D1563791

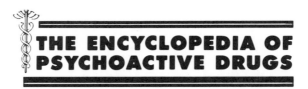

THE ENCYCLOPEDIA OF PSYCHOACTIVE DRUGS

SERIES 1

SERIES 2

DRUGS
&
PERCEPTION

GENERAL EDITOR
Professor Solomon H. Snyder, M.D.

*Distinguished Service Professor of
Neuroscience, Pharmacology, and Psychiatry at
The Johns Hopkins University School of Medicine*

•

ASSOCIATE EDITOR
Professor Barry L. Jacobs, Ph.D.

*Program in Neuroscience, Department of Psychology,
Princeton University*

•

SENIOR EDITORIAL CONSULTANT
Joann Rodgers

*Deputy Director, Office of Public Affairs at
The Johns Hopkins Medical Institutions*

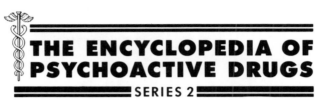

THE ENCYCLOPEDIA OF PSYCHOACTIVE DRUGS

SERIES 2

DRUGS

& PERCEPTION

WILLIAM A. CHECK

CHELSEA HOUSE PUBLISHERS
NEW YORK • PHILADELPHIA

EDITOR-IN-CHIEF: Nancy Toff
EXECUTIVE EDITOR: Remmel T. Nunn
MANAGING EDITOR: Karyn Gullen Browne
COPY CHIEF: Juliann Barbato
PICTURE EDITOR: Adrian G. Allen
ART DIRECTOR: Giannella Garrett
MANUFACTURING MANAGER: Gerald Levine

Staff for DRUGS AND PERCEPTION:

SENIOR EDITOR: Jane Larkin Crain
ASSOCIATE EDITOR: Paula Edelson
ASSISTANT EDITOR: Laura-Ann Dolce
COPY EDITOR: James Guiry
EDITORIAL ASSISTANT: Susan DeRosa
DEPUTY COPY CHIEF: Ellen Scordato
ASSOCIATE PICTURE EDITOR: Juliette Dickstein
PICTURE RESEARCHER: Villette Harris
DESIGNER: Victoria Tomaselli
DESIGN ASSISTANT: Ghila Krajzman
PRODUCTION COORDINATOR: Joseph Romano
COVER ILLUSTRATION: Linda Draper

CREATIVE DIRECTOR: Harold Steinberg

3   5   7   9   8   6   4
Library of Congress Cataloging in Publication Data

Check, William A.
  Drugs & Perception / William Check.
  p. cm.—(The Encyclopedia of psychoactive drugs. Series 2)
  Bibliography: p.
  Includes index.
  Summary: Explains the effects of psychoactive drugs on the senses including
such experiences as distorted self-image, paranoia, damage to the sensory organs,
and confusion of reality and illusion.
    1. Psychotropic drugs—Physiological effect—Juvenile literature. 2. Substance
abuse—Juvenile literature. 3. Perception—Juvenile literature. [1. Psychotropic
drugs—Physiological effect. 2. Substance abuse. 3. Perception.]
I. Title. II. Title: Drugs and perception. III. Series.
RM316.C48   1988   615'.788—dc19   87-29501   CIP   AC

ISBN 1-55546-214-6
    0-7910-0790-1 (pbk.)

CONTENTS

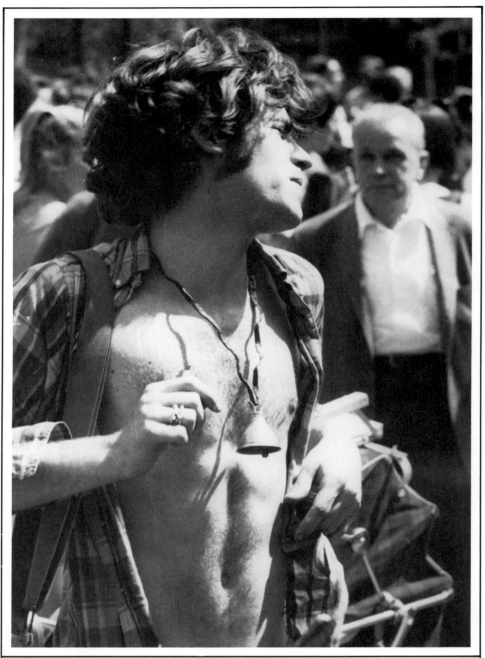

A hippie dancing at a concert during the late 1960s. During this period, the use of mind-altering drugs became commonplace, with consequences that are still being felt decades later.

In the Mainstream
of American Life

One of the legacies of the social upheaval of the 1960s is that psychoactive drugs have become part of the mainstream of American life. Schools, homes, and communities cannot be "drug proofed." There is a demand for drugs — and the supply is plentiful. Social norms have changed and drugs are not only available—they are everywhere.

But where efforts to curtail the supply of drugs and outlaw their use have had tragically limited effects on demand, it may be that education has begun to stem the rising tide of drug abuse among young people and adults alike.

Over the past 25 years, as drugs have become an increasingly routine facet of contemporary life, a great many teenagers have adopted the notion that drug taking was somehow a right or a privilege or a necessity. They have done so, however, without understanding the consequences of drug use during the crucial years of adolescence.

The teenage years are few in the total life cycle, but critical in the maturation process. During these years adolescents face the difficult tasks of discovering their identity, clarifying their sexual roles, asserting their independence, learning to cope with authority, and searching for goals that will give their lives meaning.

Drugs rob adolescents of precious time, stamina, and health. They interrupt critical learning processes, sometimes forever. Teenagers who use drugs are likely to withdraw increasingly into themselves, to "cop out" at just the time when they most need to reach out and experience the world.

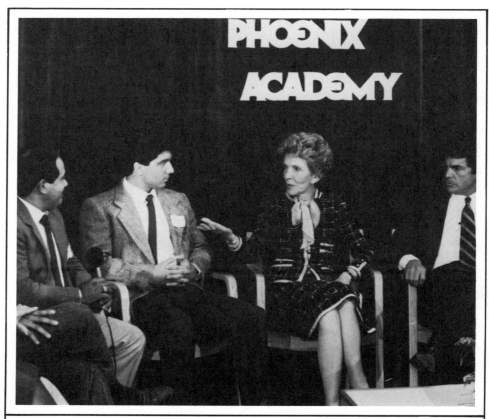

During the 1980s, First Lady Nancy Reagan spearheaded a national campaign to alert the public to the dangers of drug abuse. She is shown here at Phoenix Academy, a drug rehabilitation school.

Fortunately, as a recent Gallup poll shows, young people are beginning to realize this, too. They themselves label drugs their most important problem. In the last few years, moreover, the climate of tolerance and ignorance surrounding drugs has been changing.

Adolescents as well as adults are becoming aware of mounting evidence that every race, ethnic group, and class is vulnerable to drug dependency.

Recent publicity about the cost and failure of drug rehabilitation efforts; dangerous drug use among pilots, air traffic controllers, star athletes, and Hollywood celebrities; and drug-related accidents, suicides, and violent crime have focused the public's attention on the need to wage an all-out war on drug abuse before it seriously undermines the fabric of society itself.

The anti-drug message is getting stronger and there is evidence that the message is beginning to get through to adults and teenagers alike.

war on drug abuse before it seriously undermines the fabric of society itself.

The anti-drug message is getting stronger and there is evidence that the message is beginning to get through to adults and teenagers alike.

The Encyclopedia of Psychoactive Drugs hopes to play a part in the national campaign now underway to educate young people about drugs. Series 1 provides clear and comprehensive discussions of common psychoactive substances, outlines their psychological and physiological effects on the mind and body, explains how they "hook" the user, and separates fact from myth in the complex issue of drug abuse.

Whereas Series 1 focuses on specific drugs, such as nicotine or cocaine, Series 2 confronts a broad range of both social and physiological phenomena. Each volume addresses the ramifications of drug use and abuse on some aspect of human experience: social, familial, cultural, historical, and physical. Separate volumes explore questions about the effects of drugs on brain chemistry and unborn children; the use and abuse of painkillers; the relationship between drugs and sexual behavior, sports, and the arts; drugs and disease; the role of drugs in history; and the sophisticated drugs now being developed in the laboratory that will profoundly change the future.

Each book in the series is fully illustrated and is tailored to the needs and interests of young readers. The more adolescents know about drugs and their role in society, the less likely they are to misuse them.

Joann Rodgers
Senior Editorial Consultant

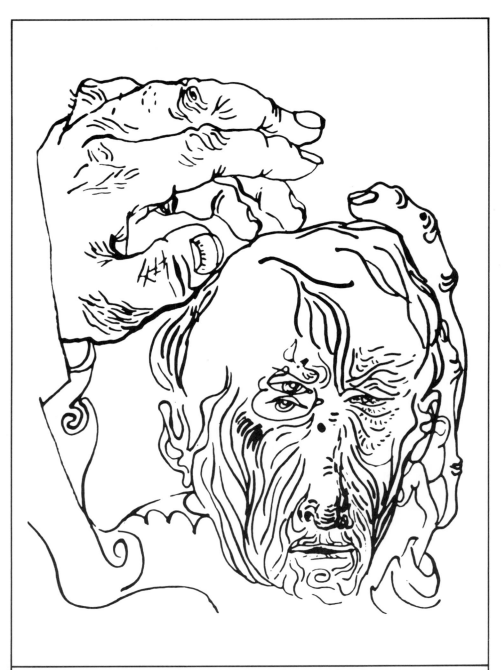

This drawing was made by a professional artist after he recovered from an LSD experience. It graphically illustrates some of the ways hallucinogens can distort a person's visual and spatial perceptions.

INTRODUCTION

The Gift of Wizardry
Use and Abuse

JACK H. MENDELSON, M.D.
NANCY K. MELLO, Ph.D.
Alcohol and Drug Abuse Research Center
Harvard Medical School—McLean Hospital

Dorothy to the Wizard:
"I think you are a very bad man," said Dorothy.
"Oh no, my dear; I'm really a very good man; but I'm a very bad Wizard."
—from THE WIZARD OF OZ

Man is endowed with the gift of wizardry, a talent for discovery and invention. The discovery and invention of substances that change the way we feel and behave are among man's special accomplishments, and, like so many other products of our wizardry, these substances have the capacity to harm as well as to help. Psychoactive drugs can cause profound changes in the chemistry of the brain and other vital organs, and although their legitimate use can relieve pain and cure disease, their abuse leads in a tragic number of cases to destruction.

Consider alcohol — available to all and yet regarded with intense ambivalence from biblical times to the present day. The use of alcoholic beverages dates back to our earliest ancestors. Alcohol use and misuse became associated with the worship of gods and demons. One of the most powerful Greek gods was Dionysus, lord of fruitfulness and god of wine. The Romans adopted Dionysus but changed his name to Bacchus. Festivals and holidays associated with Bacchus celebrated the harvest and the origins of life. Time has blurred the images of the Bacchanalian festival, but the theme of

13

drunkenness as a major part of celebration has survived the pagan gods and remains a familiar part of modern society. The term "Bacchanalian Festival" conveys a more appealing image than "drunken orgy" or "pot party," but whatever the label, drinking alcohol is a form of drug use that results in addiction for millions.

The fact that many millions of other people can use alcohol in moderation does not mitigate the toll this drug takes on society as a whole. According to reliable estimates, one out of every ten Americans develops a serious alcohol-related problem sometime in his or her lifetime. In addition, automobile accidents caused by drunken drivers claim the lives of tens of thousands every year. Many of the victims are gifted young people, just starting out in adult life. Hospital emergency rooms abound with patients seeking help for alcohol-related injuries.

Who is to blame? Can we blame the many manufacturers who produce such an amazing variety of alcoholic beverages? Should we blame the educators who fail to explain the perils of intoxication, or so exaggerate the dangers of drinking that no one could possibly believe them? Are friends to blame — those peers who urge others to "drink more and faster," or the macho types who stress the importance of being able to "hold your liquor"? Casting blame, however, is hardly constructive, and pointing the finger is a fruitless way to deal with the problem. Alcoholism and drug abuse have few culprits but many victims. Accountability begins with each of us, every time we choose to use or misuse an intoxicating substance.

It is ironic that some of man's earliest medicines, derived from natural plant products, are used today to poison and to intoxicate. Relief from pain and suffering is one of society's many continuing goals. Over 3,000 years ago, the Therapeutic Papyrus of Thebes, one of our earliest written records, gave instructions for the use of opium in the treatment of pain. Opium, in the form of its major derivative, morphine, and similar compounds, such as heroin, have also been used by many to induce changes in mood and feeling. Another example of man's misuse of a natural substance is the coca leaf, which for centuries was used by the Indians of Peru to reduce fatigue and hunger. Its modern derivative, cocaine, has important medical use as a local anesthetic. Unfortunately, its increasing abuse in the 1980s clearly has reached epidemic proportions.

The purpose of this series is to explore in depth the psychological and behavioral effects that psychoactive drugs have on the individual, and also, to investigate the ways in which drug use influences the legal, economic, cultural, and even moral aspects of societies. The information presented here (and in other books in this series) is based on many clinical and laboratory studies and other observations by people from diverse walks of life.

Over the centuries, novelists, poets, and dramatists have provided us with many insights into the sometimes seductive but ultimately problematic aspects of alcohol and drug use. Physicians, lawyers, biologists, psychologists, and social scientists have contributed to a better understanding of the causes and consequences of using these substances. The authors in this series have attempted to gather and condense all the latest information about drug use and abuse. They have also described the sometimes wide gaps in our knowledge and have suggested some new ways to answer many difficult questions.

One such question, for example, is how do alcohol and drug problems get started? And what is the best way to treat them when they do? Not too many years ago, alcoholics and drug abusers were regarded as evil, immoral, or both. It is now recognized that these persons suffer from very complicated diseases involving deep psychological and social problems. To understand how the disease begins and progresses, it is necessary to understand the nature of the substance, the behavior of addicts, and the characteristics of the society or culture in which they live.

Although many of the social environments we live in are very similar, some of the most subtle differences can strongly influence our thinking and behavior. Where we live, go to school and work, whom we discuss things with — all influence our opinions about drug use and misuse. Yet we also share certain commonly accepted beliefs that outweigh any differences in our attitudes. The authors in this series have tried to identify and discuss the central, most crucial issues concerning drug use and misuse.

Despite the increasing sophistication of the chemical substances we create in the laboratory, we have a long way to go in our efforts to make these powerful drugs work for us rather than against us.

The volumes in this series address a wide range of timely questions. What influence has drug use had on the arts? Why do so many of today's celebrities and star athletes use drugs, and what is being done to solve this problem? What is the relationship between drugs and crime? What is the physiological basis for the power drugs can hold over us? These are but a few of the issues explored in this far-ranging series.

Educating people about the dangers of drugs can go a long way towards minimizing the desperate consequences of substance abuse for individuals and society as a whole. Luckily, human beings have the resources to solve even the most serious problems that beset them, once they make the commitment to do so. As one keen and sensitive observer, Dr. Lewis Thomas, has said,

> There is nothing at all absurd about the human condition. We matter. It seems to me a good guess, hazarded by a good many people who have thought about it, that we may be engaged in the formation of something like a mind for the life of this planet. If this is so, we are still at the most primitive stage, still fumbling with language and thinking, but infinitely capacitated for the future. Looked at this way, it is remarkable that we've come as far as we have in so short a period, really no time at all as geologists measure time. We are the newest, youngest, and the brightest thing around.

DRUGS
&
PERCEPTION

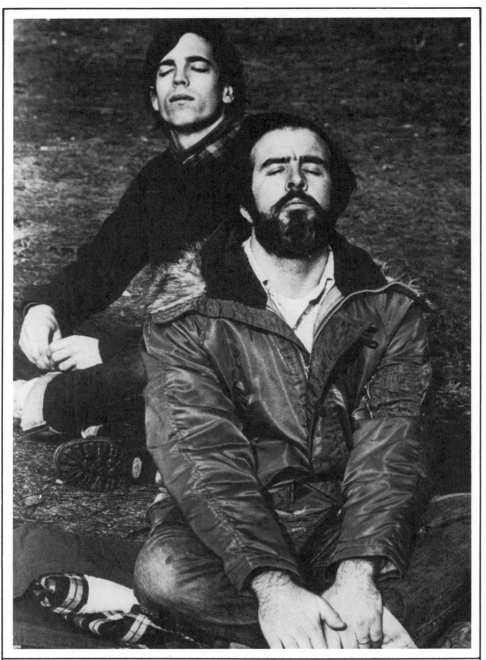

Young business executives do yoga exercises as part of a stress-reduction program. Yoga and other forms of meditation create altered states of consciousness without distorting sensory perceptions.

CHAPTER 1

KEEPING IN TOUCH
WITH THE WORLD

Most of us have taken part in a simple experiment that clearly defines the role of smell and taste in our enjoyment of food. A friend blindfolds you, holds your nose shut, and feeds you small bits of food asking you to identify what each food is. Anyone who has not tried this test might think that it would be easy to distinguish the various foods by their tastes alone. It is, however, surprisingly difficult.

Turnips and potatoes, which "taste" so different, are practically indistinguishable when you cannot smell them. Even foods with flavors as strong as those of banana or bacon are difficult to identify when you cannot smell. The reason for this difficulty is that our perception of the flavor of food is a mixture of taste and smell, with the sense of smell able to detect a much wider and more varied range of odors. Taste, in contrast, is limited to detecting only four qualities of food — saltiness, sweetness, sourness, and bitterness. Under normal circumstances the nerve signals from the tongue and the nose reach the brain simultaneously and are automatically combined, so we are unaware of the separate messages involved in our experience of good food.

Although we will further discuss aroma and taste later in this book, this example is a good demonstration of a basic principle of the senses. What we call sensations or sensory perceptions may often seem straightforward and simple, but in reality they are almost universally complex. The sense perceptions that we take for granted reflect multiple facets of the external world, and the information we receive through the sense organs is processed by the brain in a series of complicated activities that scientists still do not completely understand.

There are so many steps required for the brain to process raw information about our external and internal world into the sensations that we are used to that there is a great chance for something to go awry. In fact, what is surprising is how accurate sensations are under normal circumstances in a healthy person. But perception is a sensitive process, and it does not take much of a deviation from normal circumstances or complete health to distort it. For example, many of us, when extremely tired, have seen flashing lights or heard imaginary voices.

Another alteration that can distort perception is the taking of drugs. Most drugs taken for medicinal purposes do not produce sensory changes, mainly because prior to their approval by the government they have been tested for undesired or disorienting effects. Although some drugs can cause a ringing in the ears or a blurring of vision these side effects are generally mild and disappear when the patient stops taking the medicine.

The same cannot be said of "recreational" chemicals that are deliberately taken to alter mood or distort our view of the world. Marijuana, LSD (lysergic acid diethylamide), cocaine, and many other illicit psychoactive substances act on the brain to interfere with the normal functioning of sensation. And because the entire process of sensory perception relies on chemical activity in the brain, it should not be surprising that mind-altering chemicals can distort sensations.

To illustrate how sensory perception relies on chemical activity, take the example of smell and taste that we discussed earlier. Foods send off molecular vapors that the nose perceives as odors. Once in the mouth, food releases water-soluble chemicals that interact with special cells on the tongue to produce true tastes. Recognition by the nose of a chemical aroma or detection by the tongue of a chemical taste causes chemical signals to travel from the sensory receptor to the brain.

Once in the brain, the message sets off many more chemical reactions. Intricate nerve pathways coordinate their activity via multiple chemical signals until an intelligible sensation is produced. At that point, other chemical monitors allow the sensation to rise to the conscious brain, where we become aware of it.

With such a multiplicity of chemical transmissions required for even the simplest information about the world to reach our thinking mind, it is no wonder that many chemicals can alter the process. Scientists understand how some mind-altering drugs act. With others, the mechanism remains a mystery.

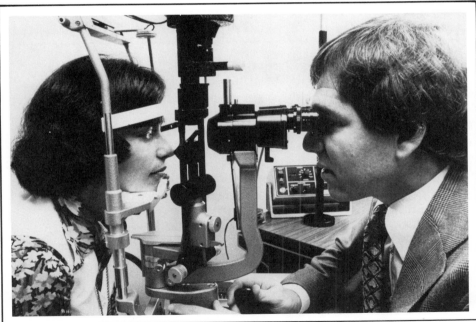

An ophthalmologist uses a laser beam to treat a form of vision impairment associated with diabetes. Sight is the most important of the special senses, and its loss the most difficult to compensate for.

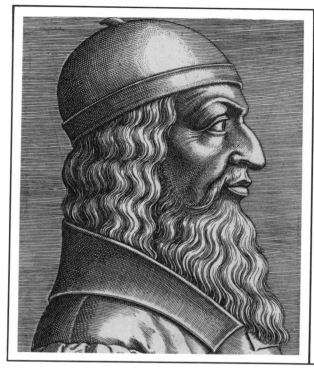

A portrait of Aristotle, the classical Greek philosopher (384–322B.C.). The five special senses of sight, hearing, taste, smell, and touch were recognized during his time. Since then, as many as 15 more have been identified.

Some illicit drugs have the ability to distort perceptions permanently after they have been taken only a few times. Glue sniffing carries this hazard. Others are more like medicines — their distortion of the senses wears off within a few hours. Unfortunately, the user typically craves a return to the altered state of perception induced by the drug. This pattern of drug abuse often leads to addiction.

Although some illicit psychoactive drugs strongly affect perception, others have their greatest effects on mood or emotion. The opiates are probably the most widely used addictive drugs that fall into this category. But many drugs of abuse affect both the emotional state and the sensory perception of the user.

Before turning to the various classes of psychoactive drugs and describing what types of distortions of reality each can cause, it is necessary to have a rudimentary understanding of how the process of normal perception works. This includes each of the classical sensations, those senses that have been known since the days of the Greek philosopher Aristotle as *special senses*—sight, hearing, taste, smell, and touch.

Since Aristotle's day, as many as 15 additional senses have been identified. They include a sense of weight, a sense of position of the body, and a sense of the degree of bending of joints. Many of these are proprioceptive senses, that is, they deal with stimuli arising from within the organism. Three physical senses that are not included in the five special senses but that nonetheless provide us with important information about the external world and about our relation to that world are the senses of time, motion, and balance.

There are also numerous psychological senses or perceptions that are disturbed by illicit drugs. These "internal sensations" primarily comprise the sense of self or self-worth, a sense of power, and a sense of well-being. Although they are not, strictly speaking, "senses," the perceptions of one's self in relation to the world are an extremely important part of each person's relationship to reality, and disturbances of these internal sensations can be another side effect of drug abuse.

Before launching into definitions, distinctions, or descriptions, it is important to state clearly one crucial conclusion that follows from all work on addictive psychoactive drugs: Most of these drugs do drastically alter our perceptions both of physical stimuli from the outside world and of the way we see ourselves as persons.

If there is an exception, it is drugs that sedate the brain. These substances include alcohol as well as barbiturates and other sleeping pills. Sedatives, especially alcohol, are potentially drugs of abuse. But they do not stimulate the mind to new and unusual perceptions or offer false reassurance to the sense of self-worth. They are mind-numbing, or, in scientific terms, they are central nervous system depressants. Initially alcohol may seem to boost the ego and the imagination, because a small amount of alcohol depresses inhibitions. But any further drinking sedates the rest of the brain as well, leading to gradual loss of speech, movement, imagination, thought, and finally, conciousness. Because alcohol and other sedative drugs deaden the senses rather than stimulate them, they are not discussed in this book.

Psychoactive drugs distort one's perception of reality. Many produce hallucinations. They can disorient the senses and the personality. The distortions and disorientation can be, at best, frightening. In some instances they can be permanent, as is the case with the flashbacks following long-term use of LSD. Many of these substances lead to addiction, either physical or psychological. In extreme situations, they can even cause psychotic breakdowns.

Each psychoactive substance carries with it the potential for causing temporary loss of contact with reality in one way or another. The altered states it produces can seem seductive, but each time the user escapes from reality, he runs the risk of not reestablishing contact.

The Special Senses: How They Work

Although there are great differences in the way we apprehend various types of sensory information about our world, one principle underlies all physical perceptions: They are all ways of translating energy into sensations. Sight results from detecting and interpreting electromagnetic radiation. Sound consists of pressure waves traveling through the air. Smell and taste are produced by highly energetic molecules interacting with special receptors on the tongue or in the nose. The feeling of touch is a result of direct application of mechanical energy. When we experience heat or cold, we are sensing differences in thermal energy between an object and our skin.

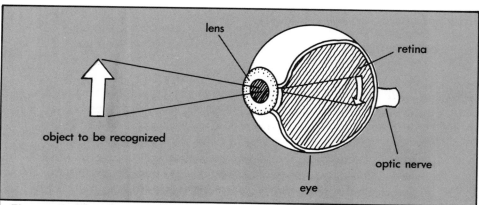

Figure 1: The Lens and Retina. The lens of the eye focuses patterns of light onto the retina. Initially, the image is reversed from top to bottom and from right to left.

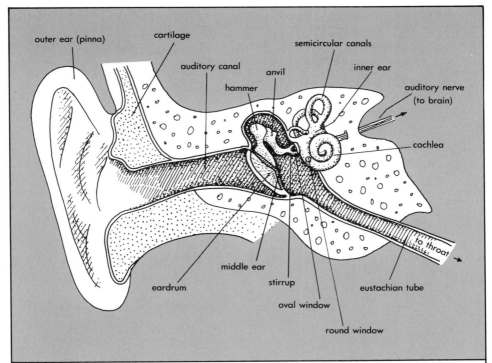

Figure 2: The External, Middle, and Inner Ear. *The sensation of hearing occurs when air pressure variations are routed to the cochlea and are translated into patterns of neural activity.*

What is unique to each mode of physical perception is the form in which the energy is packaged, the way a special sense organ perceives the energy, and the interpretation of that information in the brain.

Sight is one of the most important of the human senses. It is probably the one sense whose loss is most difficult to compensate for. Sight is the perception and interpretation of packets of electromagnetic energy called photons. Humans can perceive only those photons that fall in a special energy range. The spectrum of electromagnetic waves includes not only light but also X rays, radio waves, microwaves, ultraviolet radiation, and infrared radiation. These types of electromagnetic radiation all have characteristic wavelengths. Visible light is a narrow band that lies between the ultraviolet and infrared bands, presumed to be so because our sun emits 40% of its radiation in that range.

In a narrow technical sense, "seeing" refers to the process by which photons in the visible range of energy interact with the surface of the eye. Light enters the eye through the pupil, goes through the lens (which focuses it just as a microscope does), and registers on the retina at the rear of the eye.

The retina is composed of densely crowded cells that are sensitive to light. When a photon makes an impact on a retinal cell, that cell sends a message to the brain. The optical lobe of the brain receives these messages from the retina and interprets and coordinates them into a picture of the external world.

The two classes of light-sensitive cells on the retina are called rods and cones. Combinations of stimulation of rods and cones provide color vision. Only three colors are encoded by the retinal cells: red, green, and blue. From these three types of color messages, the brain is able to reconstruct any of a wide variety of shades of color.

Using the signals coming from the eye, the brain carries out a complex set of activities necessary to make sense of what is registering on the retina. Images are stored so that changes in size over time can be interpreted as motion. Images are compared to a databank of stored shapes to decide what — or who — you are seeing. Visual clues are consulted to decide which objects are near and which are farther away, irrespective of their size.

Hearing depends on the reverberations of pressure waves in the air against the loosely stretched flap of skin we call the eardrum, or tympanum. As the eardrum is stimulated, it produces vibrations in a set of three small bones behind it, which in turn generate waves in the liquid contained in a coiled tube, the cochlea. Waves in the cochlear fluid cause movement of hairs attached to nerve cells in the cochlea, and those hairs stimulate the nerve cells to send signals to the brain.

Of course, that does not really explain why we hear what we hear in just the way that we hear it. Much of that is done in the specialized brain areas called the auditory lobes. Certainly stereo sound depends on the brain's combining in the correct way slightly different sound messages from the two ears. Stereo sound gives us a clue to where the source of a sound is located.

Another complex function of hearing is differentiation between music and noise. This action varies from person to person, and even the same person will respond differently to different sounds at different times. Enjoyment of music is one sensation that is very much influenced by the mood changes brought about by psychoactive drugs.

As we all know, *smell* is located in the nose. Odoriferous substances give off vaporous molecules into the air. These molecules interact with special nerve-cell receptors in the nose and stimulate them to signal the brain.

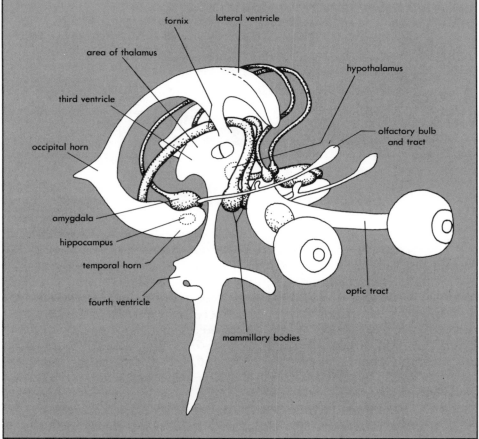

Figure 3: The Olfactory Bulb. *Nerve fibers carry sensations of smell from the olfactory bulb, a long outgrowth of the brain, to several regions in the lower, more primitive part of the forebrain.*

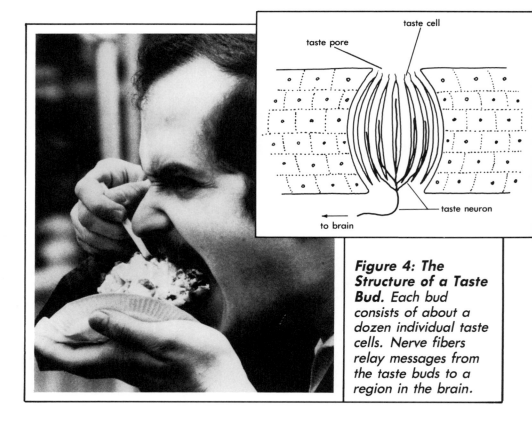

Figure 4: The Structure of a Taste Bud. *Each bud consists of about a dozen individual taste cells. Nerve fibers relay messages from the taste buds to a region in the brain.*

But how can we detect such a large variety of olfactory stimuli? Surely our nose does not contain a different set of receptors for every possible odor-carrying molecule? Current research suggests that there are seven classes of smell receptors and that a large spectrum of smells can be generated by varying interactions within these seven classes.

Taste is detected by special receptors called taste buds on the surface of the tongue. There are four types of taste buds, and they tell us whether foods (and other substances) are salty, sweet, bitter, or sour. Taste buds for each quality are distributed in special places — bitterness at the rear of the tongue, sweetness at the tip, and saltiness and sourness on the sides.

Taste used to be considered a straightforward sensation: A taste bud detected a flavor, and it sent a signal to the brain. Newer experiments have showed, however, that the same set of taste buds can respond to different flavors, each in a different way. Therefore, the brain must play a role in the processing of taste. In addition, we know that taste is combined with smell in evaluating foods.

Touch is a remarkably varied sensation. Sensors in the skin can discriminate among several types of touch, such as simple contact, pressure (dullness), heat loss (cold), heat gain (hot), and pain (sharpness). All sensors send a nerve impulse to the brain when they are stimulated. But each sensor responds to a different kind of stimulation.

In most situations, we take accurate perception for granted. But because perception is such a complicated process, situations can be devised in which the senses are confused. We will discuss this perceptual trickery in the next chapter.

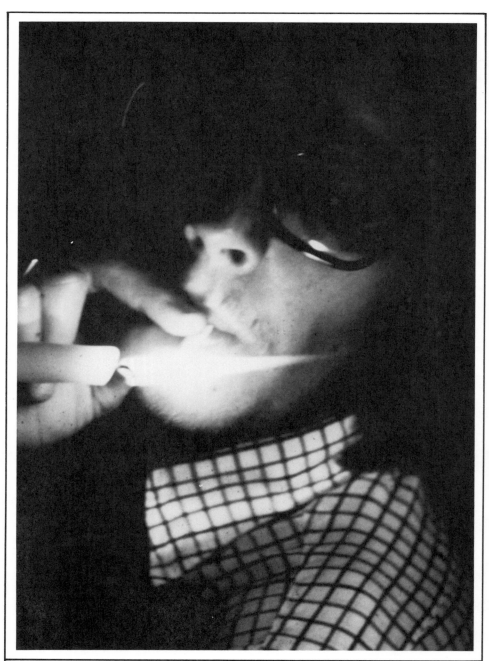

A young drug user lights up a marijuana cigarette. Marijuana is a mild hallucinogen, meaning that it distorts sensory perceptions. The effects of this drug on the sense of hearing are particularly acute.

CHAPTER 2

FOOLING THE SENSES

Trying to identify familiar foods by taste alone while some-one is holding one's nose is one way to fool the senses. Various types of optical illusions demonstrate how easy it is to trick our sense of sight. One of the most common and most obvious is the motion picture. Though it may seem that we are seeing motion, we all know that a motion picture is actually a series of still photographs passing before our eyes at a rapid rate.

Another principle of vision — that eyes move faster along horizontal lines than along vertical lines — makes it difficult to draw a perfect square freehand. Draw the best square you can. Turn it sideways. It will look too high. If you draw a perfect square with a ruler, your brain will tell you that it is too tall.

Books have been filled with descriptions of optical illusions such as these. Because the sense of sight is so complex and depends on so many supporting clues in the environment and so much processing in the brain, it is most easily fooled. Perhaps that is why, when we discuss the strongest hallucinogenic drugs, we will find that visual hallucinations are particularly common.

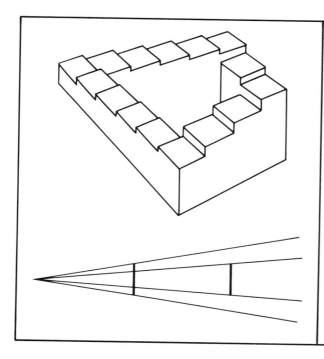

Figure 5: Optical Illusions. Top: It is impossible to tell whether the steps in this "staircase that never ends" are going up or down. Bottom: At first glance, it looks as if the parallel lines in this figure are of different lengths; in fact, the lengths are the same.

Auditory hallucinations and delusions (hearing voices) are features of the complex mental illness known as schizophrenia. In patients suffering from this illness, certain regions of the brain voluntarily — without any prompting from outside — initiate voice messages. It is highly likely that this spontaneous auditory information is the result of chemical imbalances in the brain.

Drugs are available that affect the brain chemicals thought to be disturbed in schizophrenics. These drugs moderate schizophrenic symptoms, and auditory hallucinations in particular.

As one would expect, certain hallucinogenic drugs are also capable of stimulating a person to hear imaginary voices.

The dependence of smell on complex chemical interactions was demonstrated by a medical report published a few years ago concerning a man who suddenly developed a condition called dysgeusia. Dysgeusia refers to a gross disturbance of the sense of smell. All food began to smell rotten to the man. This was most unfortunate, because he was a cook. He could no longer cook and had difficulty eating.

After the man had visited many doctors, a specialist at the National Institutes of Health finally tracked down the source of his problem. The man had an imbalance of the element nickel in his body. With restoration of the correct nickel concentration in his tissues, the problem disappeared.

The dependence of correct functioning on the senses is dramatically illustrated by experiments in which people are deprived of all sensory input, a situation called sensory deprivation. For instance, a person might be totally wrapped in a bodysuit, with blacked-out goggles over his eyes, covers over his ears, and oxygen provided through a mask so that no scents reach his nose.

After a time in this state, bizarre delusions and visual illusions often result. These hallucinations occur without the subject's losing total contact with reality, as a schizophrenic often does. Visual hallucinations, often in vivid color, are quite prominent. Complex images may be "seen." In one study, subjects were provided with only dim light in which no shapes could be discerned. One person reported "a procession of squirrels with sacks over their shoulders marching across a snow field."

A period of sensory deprivation can also produce a feeling of depersonalization and loss of body image. The arms can be dissociated from the body, or the body may seem to be floating in the air. To some people this experience is quite frightening.

What is important to realize is that such effects are similar to those experienced with many illicit drugs. The parallel emphasizes that psychoactive chemicals grossly distort the user's contact with reality, just as the highly abnormal conditions of sensory deprivation do. That is why psychoactive chemicals produce alterations in sensory perceptions and self-perception ranging from mild to severe.

Proprioceptive Senses

Special senses mediate between the external world and our internal world. These proprioceptive senses gather signals from inside the body to provide us with information about where we stand—literally—in relation to the external world. Two of these proprioceptive senses — balance and motion — are based on a complicated set of three tubes called the semicircular canals located in the inner ear. These canals are filled with a fluid that sloshes back and forth as we start and stop moving or change the direction in which we are moving, thus providing us with information about motion. It is comparatively easy to fool your sense of motion. If you spin around in place rapidly for several seconds, then stop suddenly, you will feel as though you are still moving. This is because the fluid has not settled down yet and is still sending the brain motion messages.

When information about movement from the canals is combined with information about position from other parts of the body, the result is our complex and vital sense of balance. Many disturbances of balance result from confusing or contradictory sensations arriving in the brain. Seasickness and vertigo are two examples of this phenomenon. Another is the space sickness experienced by astronauts. The brain finds it difficult to interpret motion signals in the absence of information about gravity, which is absent in space.

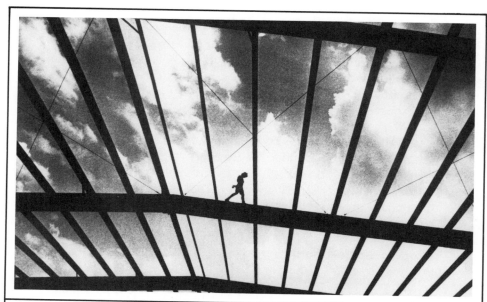

A construction worker high atop a steel scaffold. The proprioceptive sense of balance is based on a complicated set of three tubes called the semicircular canals, which are located in the inner ear.

Kinesthesia is a proprioceptive sensation that is also related to motion. It tells us more about what our body is doing to create the motion, where the various parts of our body are, and how they are moving. Kinesthesia is based on stimuli from sensors located in muscles, tendons, and joints and stimulated by bodily movements, muscular contractions, and muscular tensions.

Finally, we have the sense of *time*. Very little is known about how this internal sense operates. No internal clock has been found in humans. Our bodies do, however, undergo chemical changes throughout the day and night, and these changes have been linked to a mysterious organ in the brain called the pineal gland. The pineal gland may control hibernation in frogs and lizards, but its function in humans is still a mystery. Certainly it does not control our subjective sense of the passage of time. Under certain circumstances some people can accurately judge time intervals. But we are all familiar with expressions about the subjectivity of time passage, such as "Time flies when you're having fun." In fact, whether a person is having a good time or is bored does affect his estimate of a length of time.

Like the special senses, the proprioceptive senses are also subject to distortion by psychoactive drugs.

Alterations in the sense of time passage while under the influence of marijuana and loss of the sense of balance after drinking alcohol are good examples.

A Sense of Who You Are

Our sense of self results from a very complex mixture of information. It includes physical sensations, proprioceptive senses that tell us the condition of our body, our perceptions of how other people react to us, knowledge about our abilities, our emotional states, and much more.

What is most important to this discussion is that our sense of self-worth, well-being, or personal power can be profoundly affected by habitual drug taking. Distortions of reality can lead to disorientation and loss of contact with reality. We can become unsure of ourselves and where we stand in relation to other people, unsure even of something as fundamental as our ability to handle the physical demands of daily living.

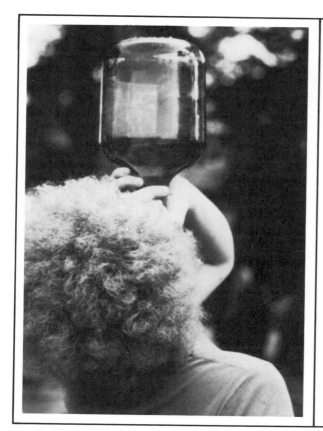

A teenager drinks red wine from the jug. The sense of balance is particularly vulnerable to the distortions caused by alcohol.

Amphetamines, for instance, can produce a falsely exaggerated sense of self. An amphetamine user's behavior can become inappropriately aggressive and exuberant in a way that is not in line with his or her true personality. That person's contacts with other people will become distorted and unrealistic.

Chronic users of methamphetamine, or "speed," can enter a state much like a severe mental illness called paranoid-schizophrenic psychosis in which their perceptions of other people become grossly distorted. The user may suffer terrifying hallucinations, mistake friends for police officers, and lash out with murderous rage at any real or imagined intrusion. The only remedy is further injection of amphetamines, which only makes the dependence worse.

A sedative medicine called Quaalude, which can no longer be manufactured legally in the United States, produces a dangerously altered sense of inner well-being in many users.

The following is a passage from a book about a man who became addicted to Quaaludes and lost contact with his wife, friends, and business. It describes the extinction of external perception produced by the drug:

> Lenny gazes off toward the blank, cold Panasonic, but his brown eyes do not see a thing. He's taken four Quaaludes and is in that part of the high where he sees absolutely nothing. It is as if he decided simply to give away an hour of his life.

Lenny liked the drug because it allowed him to escape from his self-perceived personality deficiency. Ultimately, the only way he could attain any sense of self-worth or well-being was to take several Quaaludes. He finally gave away his whole life to the drug.

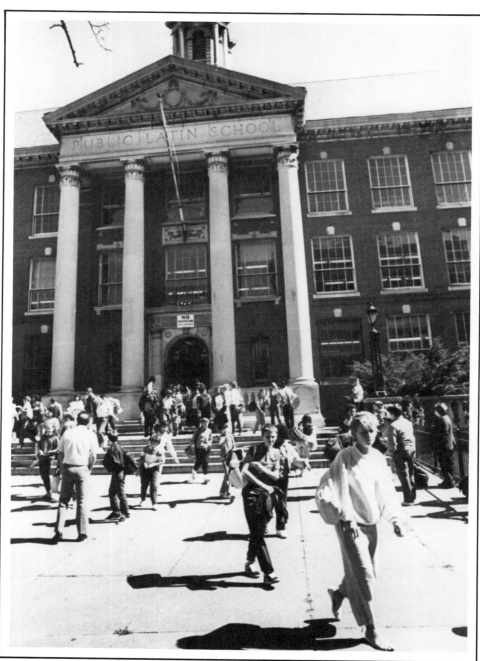

Dismissal time at the Boston Latin School, a high school renowned for its rigorous standards. Experts agree that regular marijuana use undermines the concentration necessary for high academic achievement.

CHAPTER 3

MARIJUANA

Does marijuana produce alterations in perception? If it does, are these alterations harmless? Do they make it dangerous for a person to drive or to work in a factory after smoking a marijuana cigarette? Will regular marijuana smoking dull the senses of young people, making it difficult for them to learn in school and to compete in sports? Such questions need clear answers.

We have two good sources of information on the psychoactive effects of marijuana. The first is interviews with people who have frequently smoked it and who can describe their reactions to it. The second type of data comes from laboratory experiments in which persons smoke marijuana cigarettes under controlled conditions.

In the laboratory experiments, several types of information are obtained. Scientists observe the behavior of the subjects. The subjects report on their inner feelings, sensations, and perceptions. Measurements are made of their bodily functions, such as heart rate and immune-system activity.

Ideally, scientists should now be able to make very precise statements about the effects of marijuana. That is partly true. On some topics, such as the impact of marijuana on perception and coordination, there is widespread agreement.

On other questions, however, experts are still divided. In particular, there is not yet a consensus on the extent of the long-term threat that marijuana poses to physical and psychological health.

However, all experts do agree that regular use of the drug is risky. A blue-ribbon panel of scientists convened by the government in 1982 concluded that some of the worst charges against marijuana were not yet scientifically proved. Even so, the panel cautioned that what *is* known about the effects of marijuana "justifies serious national concern." Thus, the chairman of the panel suggested, "Even if [marijuana] became generally legalized, prudence and common sense would dictate that its use [outside medicine] be discouraged."

Although the potential harm of marijuana has not yet been completely established, the years of surveys and laboratory research on the drug have indicated that the primary psychoactive effect of marijuana, the one most often reported, is that it produces mild euphoria and a state of pleasant relaxation. This research has also produced conclusive evidence that marijuana is capable of altering sensations and perceptions. While in the mind-altered state, users report many specific changes in their interactions with the outside world. Here are some of them:

- enhancement of the perception of sound and music

- striking visual images

- a drawing-out of the sense of time

- distortions in the sense of space

- loss of coordination

- alterations in sexual sensations

- an increase in sociability

- the feeling that everything is hilarious

- loss of short-term memory

- difficulty in speaking clearly

Some of these changes are interrelated. For instance, a distorted sense of space and time would impair coordination. The breakdown of inhibitions produced by marijuana, like

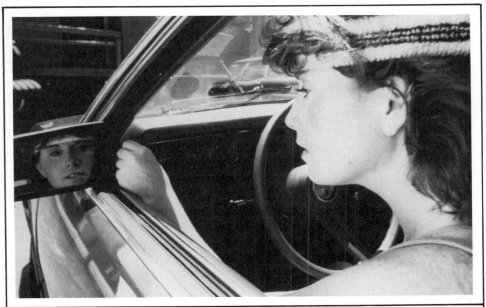

Scientific studies reveal that marijuana produces a loss of coordination and a distorted sense of time and space. Thus, driving while under the influence of this drug is dangerous and unwise.

the relaxation produced by alcohol, would increase sociability and lead to a sense of false hilarity. And a loss of the ability to think clearly would make it difficult to express ideas coherently and to understand and remember what one hears.

Based on these well-substantiated observations, we can draw some conclusions about marijuana's impact on behavior, especially on complex and demanding behaviors. These disruptions of perception, coordination, and memory have been demonstrated to be capable of the following:

- impairing the ability to operate a car safely

- making it unsafe to operate machinery

- interfering with the ability to learn in school

Of course, not all of these effects will occur in any one person during any one drug-taking episode. In fact, a person may not experience any strong alterations in mood or perception after smoking a marijuana cigarette. There are several possible reasons for this. One simple explanation could be that the THC (the psychoactive ingredient in marijuana) content of the sample is too low. But even with potent marijuana it is possible that the drug taker's psychological state may not be receptive to psychoactive changes. The setting or companions may not be conducive to relaxation. As one researcher concluded, "The mood and expectation of the subject heavily influence the psychological response to marijuana."

Another well-recognized phenomenon is the "experienced user" effect. This was seen as far back as the first laboratory study of marijuana smoking in 1968. The scientists who conducted the research found that people who had no experience smoking marijuana experienced few subjective effects or changes in perception. Experienced users, on the other hand, were more likely to report a state of euphoria and alterations in perception.

Even taking these limitations into account, it is not difficult to document the wide variety of perceptual changes

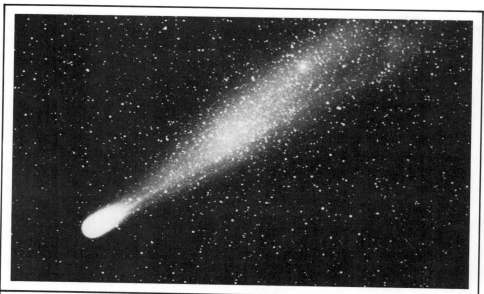

A picture of Halley's comet taken in 1986. People under the influence of marijuana have reported a number of dramatic visual hallucinations, among them exploding stars and flashes of fiery color.

that can result from marijuana smoking. One author noted that very similar effects were found both in surveys of casual users and in laboratory studies. Many of the effects involved changes in mood — the subject's internal world. But a large number of them concerned changes in perception — the user's interaction with the external world. A list of these effects (with changes in perception or senses in italics) included "*floating sensations*, depersonalization, *weakness*, relaxation, *perceptual changes in vision, hearing and touch, subjective slowing of time, loss of attention and immediate memory, difficulty of concentration*, euphoria, sleepiness . . . and *enhanced sexual performance and enjoyment*. . . . "(What are here called "floating sensations" may represent what we called "distortions in the sense of space.")

In one notable study, a questionnaire was administered to 42 randomly selected college students who had used marijuana frequently. The authors reported that "90% of the students had experienced minor changes in perception (seeing colors or objects as more intense); about half had experienced major perceptual changes (hallucinating colors or designs)." Not all researchers agree that marijuana is a hallucinogen, but there is a unanimous opinion that it can distort the user's perception of the external world.

Marijuana, Music, and Visual Perceptions

Among the many influences of marijuana on perceptions and sensation, perhaps one of the most obvious is its effect on the perception of sound, particularly music. We might have guessed this from marijuana's close association with the jazz culture. Could this be because the drug alters how music sounds? In fact, this is the case. Marijuana is well-known for its influence on auditory perception. Drug users love to listen to music under the influence of marijuana and report that their appreciation of and emotional response to musical sounds is increased after taking the drug.

What type of change does marijuana produce in the way music is perceived? That is not completely understood. No heightening of the capacity to appreciate music — including discrimination of pitch, intensity, rhythm, time, timbre, or tonal memory — has been found in people who are under the influence of marijuana. In fact, although some subjects reported that they felt their musical ability improved, in many cases it was impaired.

One clue to this puzzle of increased musical appreciation is that marijuana users report that the drug makes their hearing more acute. In extreme cases, a person under the influence of marijuana intoxication may be disturbed by the ticking of a watch or the buzzing of an insect. But laboratory testing detected no increase in hearing acuity. Perhaps, some scientists suggest, persons smoking marijuana become more aware of stimuli to which they are normally habituated. They do not hear anything new, but they are able to pay attention to more of what they hear. Thus, after smoking, a person would be aware of parts of the music that would normally be filtered out before they reached the higher brain centers.

Interestingly enough, this effect would be the opposite of a hallucination. That is, it could represent getting into greater contact with reality.

An effect that definitely represents loss of contact with reality is the production of visual images under the influence of marijuana. Although the images are not, strictly speaking, hallucinations, they are manufactured in the mind, not the external world. Colors are prominent in these images. Examples are a reddish glow, a fiery meteor, prismatic colors, or a light that is gold with blue-and-red stripes. Sparkling points of light may appear. Colors generally are brightened.

Marijuana, Space, and Time

One of the most frequently described effects of marijuana is alteration of the perception of time and space. This effect appears to be part of the overall dissociation from external reality that the marijuana user experiences. Marijuana-induced disruption in a person's perception of his surroundings was described well by one author, who wrote, "The user may have dreamlike sensations, with a free flow of ideas and distortions of time and space; a minute may seem like an hour, nearby objects may appear to be far away."

In experiments with human volunteers smoking marijuana cigarettes or taking THC orally, the distortion of time has been particularly easy to detect and to study. Subjects intoxicated with marijuana frequently state that time seems to pass slowly. This was measured directly in one study by

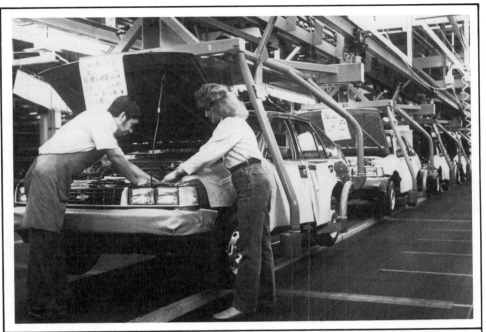

Workers on an automobile assembly line at a plant in California. There is increasing evidence that frequent marijuana use leads to lowered productivity among both white- and blue-collar workers.

asking smokers to say when they thought 20 seconds had elapsed. The smokers greatly misjudged the interval, saying 20 seconds had passed when only between 7 and 13 seconds had gone by.

In another experiment, the opposite approach was taken. Measured time intervals were used. Smokers and nonsmokers were given tasks to do during these intervals. Then they were asked how long they thought the tasks had taken. People who had not smoked thought more time had elapsed than had actually gone by. But subjects who had smoked marijuana overestimated elapsed time to an even greater extent. For instance, control subjects thought that 1 1/2 minutes seemed like 7 minutes. But marijuana smokers said it seemed like 10 minutes.

Thus, a smoker's perception of time becomes altered, out of sync with external reality. Results from both types of experiments indicate that marijuana intoxication speeds up the internal clock. Time is passing faster internally than it is externally, so external reality seems to be very slow.

It may seem a contradiction to say that the marijuana smoker's internal clock is speeded up when we have just said that marijuana seems to slow things down. But this paradox can be easily explained. Imagine a person who has taken marijuana watching someone walk across a room. She knows how long it should take. But her internal clock is going much faster than the clock on the wall. Therefore, by her internal reckoning, it seems that the person is taking forever to cross the room. The sensation is the same as when a person in real time watches a movie in slow motion.

This effect can be illustrated more vividly by an anecdote from a 1970 book by a California scientist: "Two hippies, high on pot, are sitting in Golden Gate Park in San Francisco. A jet aircraft goes zooming overhead and is gone; whereupon one hippie turns to the other and says, 'Man, I thought he'd never leave.' "

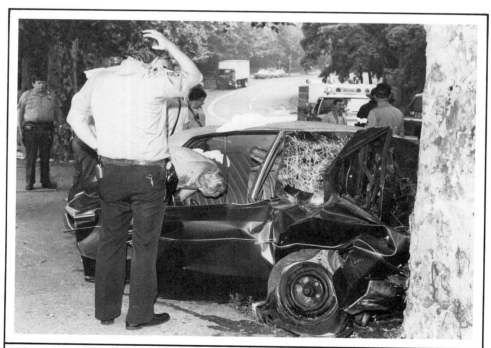

Statistics show that marijuana use contributes to the high incidence of car accidents among young people. Studies indicate that daily users of this drug have more than the average number of car accidents.

Distortions of space perception are also common and varied. Depth perception is particularly disturbed. Objects may seem either much larger or much smaller than they actually are. Walls may advance or recede. A curb may seem too high to step off. The sense of a third dimension can be lost, with people looking as though they were cut out of cardboard.

Marijuana's interference with the perception of time and space makes it difficult to perform tasks that require complex hand-eye coordination. In a pursuit rotor test, for instance, a subject is required to touch a moving spot on a computer screen with a hand-held pointer. The path taken by the light is controlled by a computer program and can be made easier or more difficult. In these types of tracking tests, people consistently score lower after they have smoked marijuana than when they are in a normal state.

Taking these alterations in time and spatial perception together, it is not surprising that complex tasks have been found to be affected by marijuana smoking. In one study, persons given THC were tested on a machine that simulated automobile driving, much like Pole Position, Spy Hunter, and other automobile-driving video games but with real-world scenes on the screen. Subjects were asked, "How long and how far do you feel you have been driving?" They overestimated both the time elapsed and the distance driven. Furthermore, errors increased with higher doses of THC.

In other studies, persons who had taken a typical social dose of marijuana lost motor coordination — their hands were unsteady, and they could not execute movements precisely.

It has been shown that the loss of coordination and judgment that occurs after using marijuana and that makes driving unsafe also makes it unsafe to fly an airplane or to operate machinery. This includes industrial equipment on a factory assembly line or construction equipment. Interference with the ability to do complex tasks, such as driving or operating machinery, can last for as long as four to eight hours after smoking a marijuana cigarette.

These observations under controlled laboratory conditions are supported by findings in the real world. There is some evidence that marijuana use contributes to the high incidence of automobile accidents among young people. Studies of highway accidents and fatalities as well as ques-

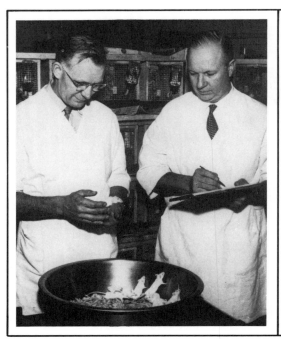

In laboratory experiments with mice, scientists found that THC stimulates an increase in testosterone immediately after it is administered but that this increased level drops off quickly thereafter.

tionnaires show that daily marijuana users have more than the average number of car accidents.

Even marijuana smokers themselves recognize that their ability to drive a car is impaired while they are intoxicated. One scientist reports this result: "We simply asked our subjects when they were high on marijuana, 'Do you think you could drive a car?' Without exception the answer from those who had really gotten high has been 'no' or 'you must be kidding.' "

Marijuana and Sexuality

One of the better-understood aspects of marijuana concerns how it affects sexual sensations. For several years researchers were puzzled by the conflict between what smokers reported and what they found in laboratory studies with animals. Marijuana users have insisted for years that the drug does wonders for their love life. However, in experiments with mice, scientists found that the substance depresses sexual desire.

In 1981, a scientist at the University of Texas solved this quandary by conducting her experiments slightly differently. She gave male animals THC, then immediately put them together with female mice. In this situation the male mice acted the way human marijuana smokers said they should. The reason: Marijuana stimulates an increase in the male sex hormone testosterone immediately after it is administered. But the increased testosterone level drops quickly. So sexual interest increases right after smoking, then soon disappears.

"I'm as guilty as other animal scientists in the last few years of neglecting what people were saying about their experiences," the scientist admitted.

The same investigator showed that the effect of marijuana on sexuality depends on how much is administered. A large dose causes an immediate dramatic drop in testosterone and a drop in sexual interest in mice. That corresponds with reports by chronic marijuana users that smoking three to five marijuana cigarettes per day impairs sexual functioning.

Marijuana and Cognitive Disturbances

Finally, there is a category of effects produced by marijuana that consists of cognitive disturbances, that is, a loss of the ability to carry out mental functions correctly. The mental functions that are affected by marijuana include memory, speech, and the ability to pay attention. We might call this class of activities "intellectual perception," because they consist of perceiving and responding to intellectual stimuli in the environment, just as physical perception consists of perceiving and responding to physical stimuli.

Marijuana's damaging effect on memory appears to be specific. It does not erase what was learned before the drug episode, but it does make it more difficult to learn while under the influence of the drug.

After smoking marijuana or ingesting THC, research subjects had difficulty performing memory tasks. Their span of attention appeared to be greatly shortened. For example, they had trouble doing moderately complex arithmetic problems, such as starting with the number 113 and alternately subtracting 7 and adding 2. In another test, subjects were taught to associate a series of numbers with colored buttons. While under the influence of marijuana they had a much harder time pressing the correct button when a number was given.

These disturbances of memory contribute to difficulty in speaking coherently. After ingesting marijuana, people become very talkative. But much of what they say does not make sense. In an early study of marijuana's effects, people who habitually smoked marijuana were recorded while speaking under the influence of the drug. Each smoker was asked to relate "an interesting or dramatic experience" in his or her life. The investigators reported that these stories were not told coherently, the subjects did not maintain a good narrative sequence, and sentences and thoughts were not expressed completely. Moreover, unrelated thoughts and facts were often allowed to intrude into the story.

When a story was read to marijuana smokers and they were asked to repeat the main points of the story back to the experimenter, many could not do it. They omitted much of the significant content of the story.

One group of investigators attributed the difficulty in telling a story to memory impairment. The problem, they said, is that "a high individual appears to have to expend more effort than when not intoxicated to remember from moment to moment the logical thread of what he is saying." The train of thought can be lost and irrelevant ideas introduced because the marijuana-intoxicated speaker forgets from one second to the next what he or she has just said.

Scientists are still working to understand how marijuana interferes with intellectual perceptions and mental activities. It can accurately be said, however, that marijuana distorts mental perceptions just as it does sensory ones. The brain of a marijuana smoker does not interpret visual messages from the outside world correctly. We might also expect it to have trouble in correctly perceiving and remembering the more complex messages contained in speech.

In addition, it is thought that memory is dependent on establishing correct time relationships among events. We have seen that marijuana distorts the sense of time. The cumulative impairment of time sense and memory would make intelligent speech difficult. As the American philosopher William James so aptly put it: "In hashish [like marijuana, a derivative of the hemp plant] intoxication there is a curious increase in the apparent time-perspective. We utter a sentence, and before the end is reached the beginning seems already to date from indefinitely long ago."

More important than how marijuana impairs intellectual perceptions and performance is the consequence of this effect. That is, it makes learning under the influence of marijuana extremely difficult. Because an increasing number of young students smoke marijuana during school hours, their learning and academic performance may be affected.

The implications for young people are extremely serious. Marijuana's distortions of perception are not just an amusement that can be called "recreational" and considered harmless. This substance can impair mental perceptions in a way that interferes with learning, impairs a young person's school career, and ultimately can damage his life and livelihood.

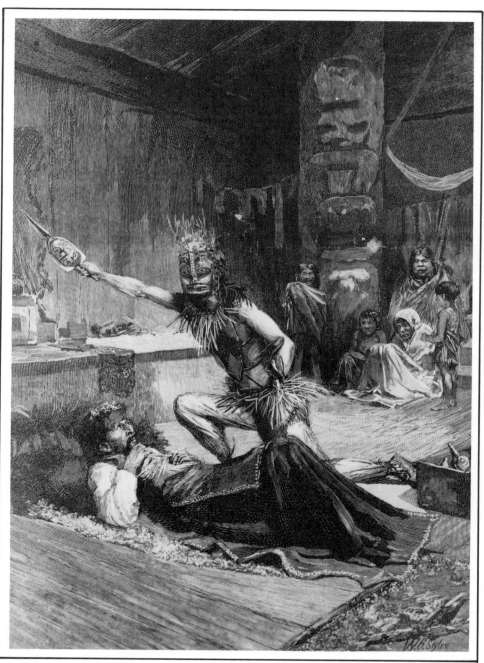

An Alaskan medicine man treating a sick person. Anthropologists have learned that some spiritual healers used natural hallucinogens to put themselves into trancelike states before ministering to the sick.

CHAPTER 4

LSD AND OTHER HALLUCINOGENS

Humans have been self-administering hallucinogenic drugs prepared from plants for several hundred years and apparently in a few societies for thousands of years. Archaeologists have uncovered signs that these substances were used as long ago as 8500 B.C. in Central America.

Historically, the use of such drugs was almost exclusively for religious and/or mystical purposes. The visions that the drugs induced were compatible with magical and primitive interpretations of the world and a belief in spirits. It was thought that use of the drugs provided insight into the foundations of the world and contact with another existence parallel to our visible one. Thus, they became the focus and facilitating agent in religious and magical rituals.

With the conquest of native tribes by Europeans during the last 500 years, use of these natural substances almost disappeared as the cultures within which the rituals arose were destroyed. In our time, however, there has been a resurgence of scientific interest in the use of natural substances for medicinal purposes. Through modern research we have become reacquainted with natural hallucinogens. Scholars have verified legends and accounts of the effects of the drugs that were found in ancient and medieval writings.

A complete list of natural hallucinogens would be quite long, for many are rather mild and used only locally. The number of truly potent plant hallucinogens that have figured in the rituals of the powerful civilizations of history is much shorter. This short list includes the following substances.

Peyote: Peyote is made from certain species of cacti found in Central and South America and in the southwestern United States. The cactus is usually prepared as dried buttons. Peyote contains the psychoactive chemical mescaline, which is one of the oldest and best-known hallucinogenic drugs and one of the most potent natural hallucinogens.

Peyote is still used by indigenous populations of Central America and the American Southwest. It is also used as part of the religious rituals of the Native American Church, a Christian religious fellowship founded in Oklahoma in 1918. The U.S. Supreme Court ruled that this use is not only legal but is protected by the U.S. Constitution's guarantee of freedom of religion. It is the only such dispensation so far granted in the United States.

Psilocybin: This is the main active ingredient in teonanacatl, the sacred mushroom of Central America. The word teonanacatl means "God's flesh" or "sacred mushrooms." It is one of the oldest known hallucinogenic preparations, with written records of its use dating back 3,000 years and other evidence suggesting that it has been used even longer. "Mushroom stones" of great antiquity have been found in Guatemala. They are stone carvings of mushrooms, the stems of which depict the head or entire figure of a god, that are at least 3,000 years old.

Mushroom-based hallucinogens became known to us with the Mexican expeditions of two scientists, R. Gordon Wasson and Valentina P. Wasson, between 1953 and 1955. They took part in several secret mushroom ceremonies and personally experienced the hallucinogenic effects of teonanacatl. Through their work it was found that the sacred mushrooms were of the *Psilocybe* and *Stropharia* genera. The hallucinogenic agent is the chemical psilocybin. LSD is a relatively recent synthetic cousin of psilocybin.

In tests conducted to measure the hallucinogenic strength of dried mushrooms, it was found that a large number were required to produce an effect. Albert Hofmann, the doctor who first synthesized LSD, tested the preparations on himself. He found that to feel any effect he had to ingest 32 dried specimens of the mushroom, a medium dose by Indian standards.

Muscimol: This is also one of the oldest hallucinogenic agents known to us. It has recently been identified with the legendary substance called Soma used by the Sanskrits 2,000 years before Christ. Muscimol is derived from the fly agaric (*Amanita*) mushroom. It is weaker than either peyote or psilocybin.

Nightshade: A group of plants used in Europe, with a high level of popularity in the Middle Ages, all belong to the Nightshade family. These were used by so-called witches to induce trances. They are weak even in relation to muscimol.

Deliriants: Another class of psychoactive natural substances found in plants that grow all over the world is the group of drugs called deliriants. What they seem to have in common, as discovered by 20th century science, is that they all interfere with a particular chemical system of the brain, the cholinergic system. Therefore, these chemicals are called anticholinergics.

Anticholinergics include the contemporary synthetic drug phencyclidine (PCP), which will be covered in Chapter 6. Natural compounds in this group, together with the plants in which they are chiefly found, are the following:

- hyoscine: Hyoscyamus niger (henbane)

- atropine: Atropa belladonna (belladonna)

- scopolamine: Datura stramonium (jimson weed, locoweed)

Most of these plants contain more than one of these compounds. The plant *Mandragora officinalis* (mandrake) contains all three.

There is some dispute about whether anticholinergic drugs are true hallucinogens. Like the synthetic anticholinergic PCP, natural drugs of this type do produce hallucinations of a disturbing character. However, they also produce a state of confusion and agitation as well as unpleasant feelings and loss of memory. The American psychopharmacologist Leo Hollister has commented about these substances, "One

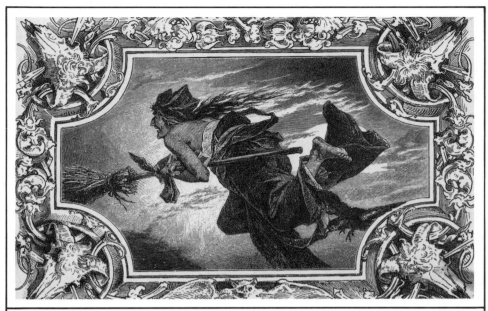

The psychoactive plants belladonna, mandrake, and henbane were often used in witchcraft because they induced wild and frenzied visions.

wonders why they are used at all, for in most cases, the experience is unpleasant or frightening."

Anticholinergics may have been the drugs that "witches" used in their gatherings. They rubbed their naked bodies with ointment containing belladonna, mandrake, and henbane. Eventually they fell into intoxicated states, with visions of flying in spirals, wild rides, and frenzied dancing. The witch's broom may have been used to simulate a horse, for riding or flying illusions.

When witches talked about their trances, they referred to long rides through the sky. Nonwitches interpreted these visions as rides taken with the Devil. Thus, even in Western Europe, hallucinations induced by drugs were interpreted in the light of magical or mystical religious thinking embedded in the culture.

It is clear from these summaries that the most potent natural hallucinogens come from the New World (Central and South America) rather than from Asia or Africa, which has been attributed to an accident of plant distribution.

To some extent, the descriptions of natural hallucinogens illuminate the effects of LSD, because LSD, mescaline, and psilocybin all belong to the same chemical family and have virtually identical effects. The chief difference is their potency, with LSD being by far the most potent hallucinogen known to date.

Hallucinogens and Perceptual Distortions

For the purposes of this chapter, it will suffice to use a simple and widely accepted definition of hallucinogens. When we use the term *hallucinogen* we refer to chemicals that, in nontoxic doses, consistently produce changes in perception, thought, and mood but seldom cause mental confusion and loss of memory.

Although this definition is accurate, it does not hint at the vivid and realistic nature of drug-induced hallucinations. In 1890 the American psychologist William James wrote of hallucinations produced by the drug experience:

> [Hallucinations] are often talked of as mental images projected outwards by mistake. But where an hallucination is complete, it is more than a mental image. An hallucination is a strictly sensational form of consciousness, as good and true as if there were a real object there. The object happens not to be there, that is all.

The German scientist A. Heffter, who isolated mescaline in 1896, gave us our first and classical account of a true hallucinogenic experience:

> Violet and green spots appear on the paper during reading. When the eyes are kept shut . . . violet and green spots which are not well defined, then come visions of carpet patterns, ribbed vaulting, etc. From time to time single dots with the most brilliant colours float across. . . . Later on landscapes, halls, architectural scenes (pillars decorated with flowers) also appear.

Heffter said that he also experienced spatial and temporal disorientation and saw vivid colors and imagery.

In 1926, the German scientist Heinrich Kluver took mescaline and provided us with the first classification scheme of visual imagery induced by drug states. Many of these types of images correspond to images described by Heffter. Kluver listed four of what he called form-constants, which were really types of shapes:

1. gratings, lattices, honeycombs, chessboards
2. cobwebs
3. funnels, tunnels, alleys, cones
4. spirals

LSD: The Prototype of Hallucinogenic Drugs

Albert Hofmann was a respected modern research chemist at Sandoz Laboratories in Basel, Switzerland. In 1943 he had a totally unexpected experience. As is the practice of traditional chemists, Hofmann tasted a tiny amount of any new

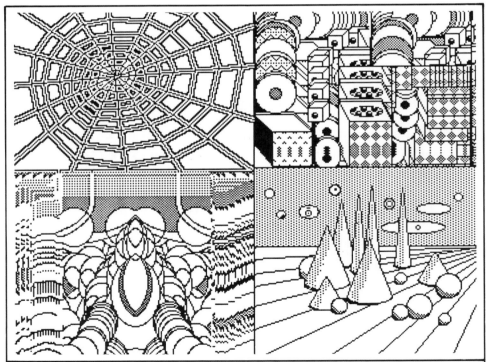

An artist's rendering of Heinrich Kluver's categories of the forms of visual images induced by drug states: cobwebs, gratings, spirals, and cones. He developed this schema after experimenting with mescaline.

chemical he made and recorded the taste as part of the catalog of the compound's properties. One day he started to feel very strange, disembodied, and restless.

Although Hofmann did not know it, he had inadvertently ushered in the modern age of psychedelic drugs. To find out which chemical had produced the effect, he proceeded to take small doses of any substance with which he could have come into contact that fateful day. After three days of sampling, he took a minute dose — 250 millionths of a gram — of a new chemical, lysergic acid diethylamide-25. Hofmann thought he was taking a conservative dose, but in fact this tiny amount was three to five times the amount of LSD needed to produce hallucinogenic effects. He wrote of his experience:

> I lost all control of time; space and time became more and more disorganized and I was overcome with fears that I was going crazy. The worst part of it was that I was clearly aware of my condition though I was incapable of stopping it.

Six hours later the trance still continued:

> [T]he perceptual distortions were still present. Everything seemed to undulate and their proportions were distorted like the reflections on a choppy water surface. Everything was changing with unpleasant, predominantly poisonous green and blue color tone. With closed eyes multihued metamorphosing fantastic images overwhelmed me. Especially noteworthy was the fact that sounds were transposed into visual sensations so that from every tone or noise a comparable colored picture was evoked, changing in form and color.

Four aspects of this experience are worth noting. One, the extremely small dose that Hofmann took produced intense hallucinogenic effects that lasted about eight hours. Two, the full range of hallucinogenic effects (especially color effects) reported by all later experimenters is present in this initial account. Three, the hallucinogenic state was definitely a mixed blessing in Hofmann's estimation. He found some of the milder effects pleasant, but some of the more extreme disorientation was definitely disturbing.

Four, Hofmann escaped with his mental status intact. But not all future LSD users were so fortunate. Many people have suffered psychotic breakdowns with just one use of this chemical, and others have, after repeated use, damaged their minds and fallen victim to the disturbing phenomenon called "flashbacks," which we will talk more about later. An important point, as two scientists experienced in research with hallucinogenic drugs have emphasized, is that "LSD is a dangerous drug and should be given to humans only under carefully controlled conditions and with experienced medical supervision."

One of the reasons for the widespread use of LSD is its relative ease of manufacture; another is its potency. In addition to being the most potent of all hallucinogenic drugs, LSD is the most studied, as well. One arbitrary scale for measuring hallucinogenic potency is in mescaline units. On this scale mescaline has a potency of 1; DMT (dimethyltryptamine), 4; psilocin (the more active form of psilocybin), 31; DOM (dimethoxy-4-methylamphetamine), 80; and LSD, 3,700. The amount of LSD that fits on the head of a pin is enough to provide a hallucinogenic experience for several people.

LSD is a synthetic chemical related in structure to the natural products psilocybin and DMT. It is also similar to a group of chemicals called ergot alkaloids, made by the fungus *Claviceps purpurea,* which grows on rye and other grains. The disease condition produced in humans who eat flour made from these plants is called ergotism. Descriptions of "devil possession" at the New England witchcraft trials of the 17th century sound very much like cases of ergotism.

Deliberate ingestion of ergot alkaloids for the purpose of religious hallucinations took place in ancient Greece during the Mysteries of Eleusis. There, for almost 2,000 years, initiates entered the portals of Eleusis to celebrate the divine gift of grain. They emerged the next day reporting trembling in the limbs, vertigo, nausea, and sweating.

Despite the long fascination of the human race with hallucinogenic drugs and the intense interest of modern scientists in these substances, we still do not have a clear understanding of how they work in the body. However, recent evidence suggests that several hallucinogens — LSD, psilocybin, mescaline, DOM, and DMT — all act by stimulating one type of receptor for a particular brain chemical called serotonin.

Moreover, there is not a clear definition or even agreement as to what constitutes hallucinogenic action. The uncertain state of research with hallucinogens is reflected in the wide variety of names given to these substances in the last 60 years. The term *phantastica* was proposed in 1924 by Louis Lewin, the "father of psychopharmacology." *Hallucinogen* was brought forward in 1954 and remains a favorite. However, one scientist objected, this term is "not ideal since it overemphasizes perceptual changes at the expense of the often more important changes in thought and mood."

Psychotomimetic was proposed in 1956, but it carries with it the unfortunate connotation that such drugs will induce in a normal subject a mental state similar to that which

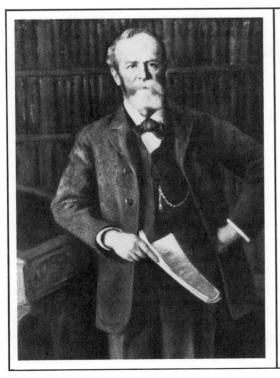

William James (1842–1910), the American psychologist and philosopher, wrote of the vivid and realistic nature of drug-induced hallucinations.

is often present in the true psychoses of many forms of mental illness. Said one researcher, "It has been pointed out several times that there are well-defined differences between mental states induced by the majority of psychotomimetic drugs and those encountered in mental illness."

The widely used term *psychedelic,* meaning "mind expanding" or "mind manifesting," was suggested in 1957 by the psychiatrist Humphrey Osmond in a letter to the British novelist and essayist Aldous Huxley.

LSD and the Psychedelic Experience

The psychedelic experience has several components. There are changes in the way the object world is perceived, which, with LSD, often involves color intensification. There may be hallucinations and illusions. Objects can change shape, either into other recognizable objects or into unrecognizable forms. Walls may appear to change in color and to move.

There may be psychic effects, cognitive disturbances such as magical and paranoid thinking, that evolve from the perceptual distortions. They can be accompanied by other elements of a thought disorder and loosening of the normal processes by which the brain associates people and things with each other.

More profound are alterations in the perception of the self and the relation of the self to the world. Many people claim to find this new perception to be a mystical or religious experience.

Perceptual changes produced by LSD are especially striking. LSD causes extraordinary changes in visual perception. For instance, users may feel that they can see the pores in other people's skin.

Soon after the drug is ingested, there are shifts in attention that may involve a sudden appreciation of the grain in a wood door rather than the door itself. For several minutes the change of state is what is impressive, with visual aspects and emotional changes gaining in intensity and frequency.

One peculiar form of perceptual distortion is called synesthesia. In synesthesia, the LSD user feels that there has been a transmutation of the senses. When someone claps his hands, the drug user feels that he can see the sound waves. An individual under the influence of LSD may see colored vibrations coming from music produced by a record player. (Hofmann alluded to this phenomenon in the account of his LSD experience quoted earlier.)

In scientific studies of many normal subjects who took LSD, sensory and emotional disturbances were common. Changes can occur in any of the senses and may be simply a distortion of sensation, a sensing of nonexistent phenomena, or hallucinations. Emotional changes can be in the direction of either euphoria and mania or depression and immobility.

In addition to alterations in sensory perception, LSD precipitates the loss of a sense of being a distinct person — the loss of ego or depersonalization that Hofmann described after his accidental ingestion of LSD. To many people, as to Hofmann, this can raise the nightmare of going crazy. The individual's personality seems to be divided into two parts, an observer and a participating self. The user is frequently unable to tell where his body ends and the surrounding environment begins.

The majority of subjects retain insight into their condition during the LSD experience and have almost complete recall. To many people these drastic distortions of perception and of normal thought processes are quite frightening.

Bad Trips and Flashbacks

There are two types of adverse reactions to the LSD experience, acute toxic psychosis and flashbacks.

Acute toxic psychosis — also known as a "bad trip" — is short-lived. It occurs while the subject is under the influence of the drug. Elements of this type of acute reaction include acute paranoia, grandiose or persecutory illusions, and a panic reaction.

The origin of a bad trip is not hard to trace. Because of the action of LSD on the central nervous system, the individual sees and perceives the environment in a fundamentally different way. Many individuals describe this as a valuable experience, but many others are frightened by it. The perceptual alterations may produce panic to the point where the individual under the influence of LSD loses control of mental processes and reacts in a self-destructive manner. The use of LSD in unsupervised circumstances increases the probability of an adverse reaction. A bad trip may produce prolonged emotional disturbances in the subject, even without repeated use of the drug.

For instance, one 19-year-old man had a bad trip in which everyone looked like a meaningless body. After recovery, he continued to feel that life was meaningless and he developed a severe depression, resulting in an attempt at suicide. Ten months later, he was still significantly depressed and under psychiatric care.

Flashbacks, on the other hand, can occur within days or years of taking a dose of LSD. They may occur after one dose but are more likely to happen in a multiple user. Flashbacks occur in between one in five and one in two LSD users.

Dr. Henry David Abraham, a psychiatrist at Harvard Medical School, studied flashbacks in a group of 123 people who were walk-in admissions to a psychiatric emergency service at a Boston hospital between 1971 and 1974. Half of the subjects had experienced flashbacks for at least five years. The visual hallucinations might last as long as five months from the time of last exposure. They took three forms: perceptual distortions, heightened imagery, and recurrent, unbidden images. Flashbacks occasionally occurred after only one exposure to LSD. They were precipitated by marijuana use and often by entering a dark environment.

Flashbacks might involve acquired color confusion (not hereditary color blindness). There might be sudden flashes of color, halos around objects, or illusions of movement, especially in the peripheral vision. For example, one subject being interviewed reported that an office coffeepot appeared to slide across the windowsill when she viewed it from the corner of her eye.

A good example of a flashback phenomenon was reported by one of the first scientists working with LSD. He was bothered for months after his single LSD experience by the flashing of the telephone poles at the periphery of his vision as he commuted daily, attempting to read the morning paper.

Another example was reported by a psychiatrist who was testing a previous LSD user who was not on LSD at the time. During one test the doctor stood near the subject, measuring his pupil size, while the subject looked at a red X on the wall. Afterward, the individual being tested said, "You are

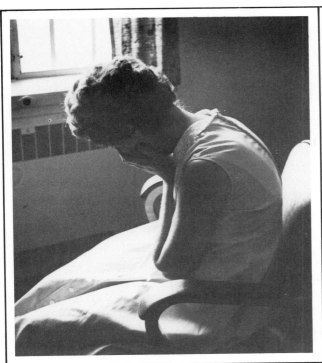

A woman sits withdrawn and depressed in a state mental hospital. Many psychologically healthy people who take LSD are vulnerable to manic or depressive reactions.

Jesus Christ on the cross." When asked what he meant, the subject explained that he was still able to see the X at the same time he was looking at the doctor. The psychiatrist called this "persistence of a mental image of what has just been seen, superimposed on an ongoing experience."

Equally as impressive as the sensory perceptual changes that occur with LSD are the alterations in the perception of the self and the relation of the self to the world.

A respected psychoanalyst has noted the similarity between the state of mind described by many people after an LSD experience and non-drug-induced insights into oneself and one's relationship to the world. Dr. Abraham Maslow conceived the idea of the "peak experience," something apart from drugs. He said that a person in peak experience feels fulfilled, creative, responsible, and at the active center of his or her life. The person in peak experience is self-determined and free of inhibitions and doubts. This feeling commonly leads to all-embracing love for everyone and everything.

When psychedelic drugs came into widespread use and reports of the spiritual aspect of the LSD trip appeared, Dr. Maslow wrote: "In the last few years it has become quite clear that certain drugs ... especially LSD and psilocybin ... often produce peak experience in the right people under the right circumstances."

LSD not only affects perceptions superficially; it appears to alter the user's very perception of his or her fundamental relationship with the universe. To some users, this feels like a religious experience. Is the outcome of the LSD trip truly mystic and religious, or is it merely a superficial delusion? A team of investigators asked 42 LSD users about their mystic experiences and how they affected the users' religious beliefs. Here is some of what they found:

- •60% said their religious feelings were changed: Half had a deeper understanding of previous religious feelings, and half experienced a change in religious thinking (though no one changed from being a believer to being agnostic or vice versa).

- •60% trusted God (or life) more; 35% trusted people more.

- •40% understood their church's doctrine better.

- •40% had less anxiety about death.

- •80% said they were more secure.

- •60% felt their personal conduct had changed for the better.

- •30% believed their moral standards had changed toward increased personal responsibility.

Based on individual interviews, the researchers concluded, "[N]o new concepts were evolved in the psychedelic experience, but new attitudes, new understandings, or new aspects of previously held concepts were elaborated."

There was greater clarity and acceptance of positive religious beliefs held by the subjects. Moreover, the investigators said, "Reinforcement of beliefs is accompanied by an increased understanding which results in a broadening, opening, and freeing of pre-existing concepts. The subjects seem to be more tolerant of other religious views."

These researchers isolated as the single most important common theme increased trust, trust based on seeing one's self more clearly and accepting that perception of the self. "Because the individual came to be on better terms with his own unconscious," they suggested, "his concept of himself was altered. Because he now saw himself differently, he found it possible to view other people and things in a different, more positive light."

Thus, we have the LSD dichotomy: It may enrich your life — at the same time leaving you open to losing your mental stability, leaving you severely depressed, and permanently altering your perceptions in a variety of frightening ways.

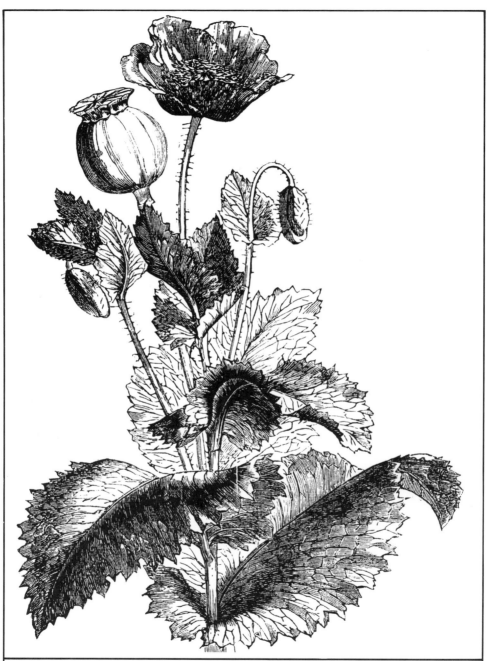

The opium poppy, from which opium, morphine, and heroin are derived. Unlike the hallucinogens, these drugs do not cause vivid and imaginative distortions of sensory perception.

CHAPTER 5

OPIATES: CREATING THE ILLUSION OF WELL-BEING

Opiates do affect the perceptions of the user, though in slightly more subtle ways than other drugs we have discussed. They produce an emotionally flat state, a condition of apathy toward the external world in which the drug taker feels neither grief nor passion. They also create an internal state of numb euphoria, which consists largely of the absence of anxiety and real-world cares. This ability to "escape" is probably what makes narcotics so attractive to certain people.

Unlike marijuana and the frankly psychedelic drugs — peyote, mescaline, and LSD — opiates do not cause vivid and imaginative delusions of sensory perception. They are not hallucinogens but narcotics.

Narcotic is both a legal and a pharmacological term, with a different meaning in each sphere. The legal definition changes arbitrarily with trends in social attitudes. It is the pharmacological definition that is relevant to a discussion of the effects of drugs on perception. Pharmacologically, a chemical is a narcotic if it produces three effects in human subjects. These three effects are pain relief, hypnosis (sleep induction), and euphoria (a feeling of intense well-being).

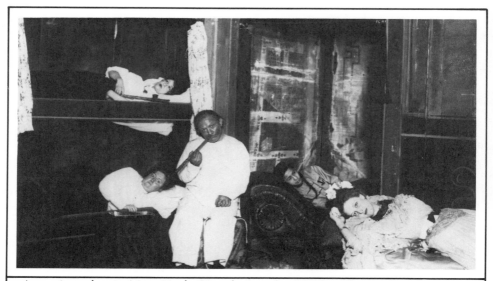

An opium den in New York City during the 1920s. The ancient Roman poet Horace wrote of the effects of opium: "A soft numbness diffuses all my inmost senses with deep oblivion."

In Western society, the term *narcotic* used in reference to drugs almost always means that class of substances designated by the term *opiates*. Opiates consist of all psychoactive substances derived from the poppy plant and all chemically modified versions of these natural substances as well as compounds made by the chemist's art that mimic the effects of natural opiates. The unifying action of all opiate compounds, both natural and synthetic, is that they act at the same sites in the brain. We will discuss this more fully later.

The definition of *narcotic* makes it clear that the opiates are not drugs that awaken the mind and make the senses more lively, creating new and imaginative perceptions of the external world. Rather, the ancient Roman poet Horace captured well the effect of opiates when he wrote, "A soft numbness diffuses all my inmost senses with deep oblivion." A key to the understanding of what opiates do to the person who takes them lies in the origin of the word. It is derived from an ancient Greek word meaning "benumbing" or "deadening." In the case of morphine or heroin, what is benumbed or deadened is both physical pain and the addict's interest in life.

In fact, the deadening effect of narcotics on the perceptions, imagination, and emotions is very marked. This phenomenon was commented on by William Burroughs, the American novelist, who used narcotics and other illicit drugs for many years. In an interview in 1969, Burroughs contrasted opiate users with the more flamboyant, and occasionally psychotic, users of psychedelic drugs. He said of opiate addicts, "They tend to be drearily sane."

Opiates and the Body

The depressing effect of opiates on emotions, imagination, and behavior is paralleled by their effects on the brain and its activity. Opiates, like alcohol, are central nervous system depressants. They decrease basic bodily functions, such as breathing and heart rate. Opiates also depress the cough re-

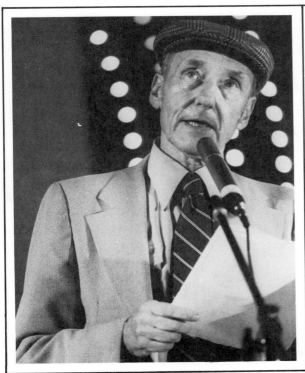

The American novelist William Burroughs abused narcotics and other illicit drugs for many years. He noted the deadening effect of narcotics on the perceptions, imagination, and emotions of the addict.

flex and reduce the muscular contractions of the intestinal wall, leading to constipation. An overdose of an opiate exaggerates these effects, leading first to nausea and vomiting and then causing unconsciousness followed by death due to cessation of respiration.

The way that opiates exert their pharmacological effects was explained in the mid-1970s with the discovery of specific brain receptors for these compounds. Both natural and laboratory-created opiates act at these sites, connecting with the receptors to achieve the desired effect.

Scientists have found that opiate receptors come in at least three varieties, and each type seems to mediate a different effect. Is it possible that one type of receptor produces pain relief and another leads to addiction? If so, will the existence of multiple opiate receptors allow science to discover a nonaddicting narcotic analgesic? The answer is not yet clear. Maybe euphoria (the addictive principle) and an-

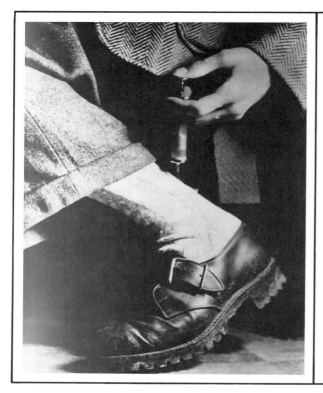

An addict injects himself with morphine. Like alcohol, this narcotic is a central nervous system depressant. Overdose can result in unconsciousness or even death.

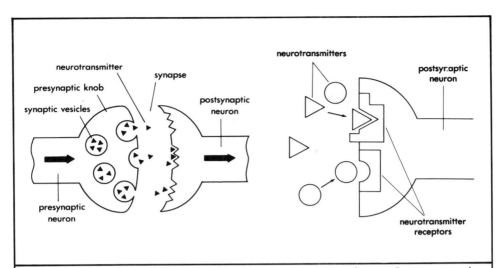

The drawing on the left shows how one neuron signals another across the synapse between them by emitting neurotransmitters. The illustration on the right shows how each kind of neurotransmitter fits only one kind of receptor on the target neuron.

algesia work through different receptors. But it is highly likely that analgesia is partly mediated via euphoria or, more generally, mood alteration. As of now, the ability to relieve pain appears to be tightly coupled to addictive potential.

Opiates and Perception

Opiates do distort perception in a number of significant ways. They affect short-term visual memory, the emotional quality of pain sensations, and the addict's emotional perception of the external world.

The effect on visual memory was found by a group of investigators in Dallas, Texas, who recently studied 467 heroin addicts who came to a Veterans Administration Medical Center for treatment of their drug habit. One type of examination given to the addicts was called a visual retention test. The subjects were shown 10 visual designs, each for 10 seconds, and immediately afterward asked to draw what they had seen.

The heroin users made more mistakes on the test than a control group of nonusers, the investigators found. They interpreted this finding as evidence of "marked perceptual disturbances" in the addicts. The researchers are now pur-

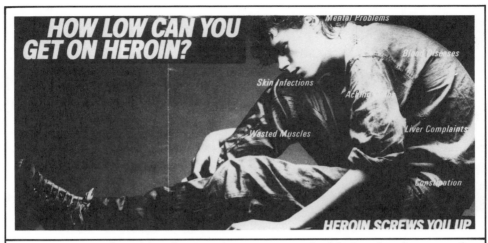

A poster produced by the British government highlights the dangers of heroin. Researchers are now pursuing the question of whether chronic heroin use produces irreversible visual-memory deficiencies.

suing the question of whether chronic heroin use produces permanent visual-memory deficiencies that persist even after drug use stops.

A more serious perceptual effect of opiates is their ability to alter the proprioceptive sense of pain. Opiates do not produce a sense of analgesia by interrupting nerve signals to the brain, as anesthetic drugs do. Rather, opiates alter the emotional quality of pain messages received in the brain. This is a subjective effect on emotional perception. As one observer said, "You're still in pain, but you don't care anymore."

This, perhaps, is the key to the widespread abuse of opiates, especially heroin. An injection of the drug makes the user indifferent to nonphysical (psychic) sources of pain in his world. With unpleasant concerns filtered out, the drug user has a good internal feeling, an illusory and temporary sense of well-being. The addict craves just this brief euphoria, this relief from anxiety and inner psychic pain. Opiates buffer the user against life's unpleasantness and troubles. One may find a heroin addict happily walking around with undetected abcessed teeth, oblivious to the acute pain and the long-term dental problem.

In general, opiates make a person oblivious to the external world, apathetic to his surroundings, and devoid of interest in all activities except getting drugs to satisfy his craving.

If you are under a physician's care, there may be nothing wrong with taking a drug for a short time to alleviate anxiety associated with real problems. However, the opiate addict does much more than that. He takes a drug that renders him oblivious to the external world and virtually nonfunctional. And he takes this drug on a long-term basis as a substitute for coping with his problems.

Here is a summary of this problem written by a doctor who treats addiction:

> In those who are feeling fatigue, worry, tension, or anxiety, the euphoriant effects afford considerable relief and may allow the individual to feel "larger than life." Although opium and the morphine alkaloids are not generally used therapeutically for mood alteration, because of their physical dependence liability, they are highly effective tranquilizers. Anxiety disappears, as do feelings of inferiority. Since the user no longer cares about life's problems in general, everything looks rosy, until the pleasurable drug effects wear off, at which time he needs a pharmacologic restoration of this euphoria with another dose.

Opiates, with their ability to release the user from his worldly cares, create a host of accompanying problems in the long run. Continued use often leads to addiction, which in turn leads to the inability to deal with life without chemical aid, certainly a most severe distortion of one's relationship to the world.

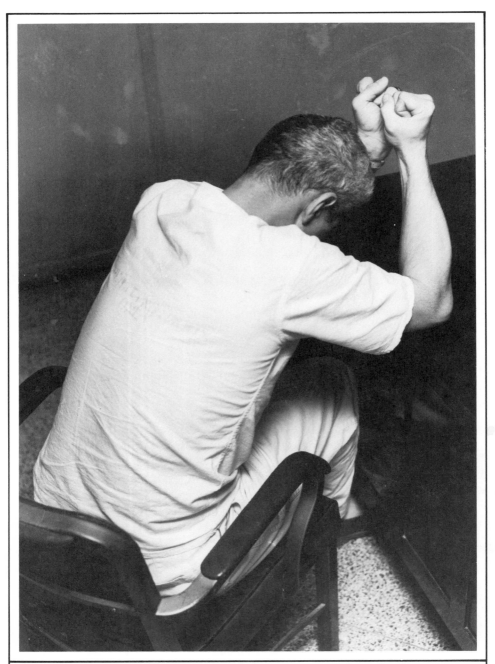

A prison inmate suffering some of the symptoms of psychosis, among them severe agitation, paranoia, and withdrawal. PCP induces these same states in users, frequently compounded by extreme violence.

CHAPTER 6

PCP: A GIANT STEP BACKWARD

As we have seen, for many centuries both European and Indian cultures used in mystic rituals a group of natural substances derived from plants of the Nightshade family, plants such as belladonna, jimsonweed, and henbane. The hallucinogenic state induced by preparations of these plants is much less attractive than trances induced by LSD, peyote, or psilocybin mushrooms. The use of these plants causes unpleasant hallucinations, disagreeable emotional sensations, and a severe hangover.

Twentieth-century chemistry has created a much more noxious and dangerous version of these anticholinergic chemicals; a substance called phencyclidine, or PCP. PCP is both unpredictable and deadly. Its complete disruption of perception, thought processes, and sense of self may be due to the fact that PCP interferes with many more brain systems than just the one served by acetylcholine. In fact, there is evidence that PCP affects practically every major brain chemical known.

Phencyclidine was originally created as an anesthetic. Ironically, it appeared to produce a state of serenity in monkeys, so it was named "Sernyl." But after this drug was used for a few years in surgery, it became clear that the drug greatly disturbed the patients' minds. Psychiatrists have even suggested that the mental state produced by PCP is so like the mental illness schizophrenia that it could be used to study how people become psychotic.

Because of these adverse effects, phencyclidine was removed from the market as a medical drug in 1965. Around 1967, PCP began to be found on the street, mostly in San Francisco. (Although phencyclidine is still marketed as a veterinary anesthetic, most of the PCP found on the street is thought to be manufactured in small-scale, illegal laboratories.) After drug takers found out how unpleasant it was, PCP could only be sold by falsely representing it as THC, mescaline, or LSD. But in the mid-1970s, PCP enjoyed a surge in popularity under its own name. A growing number of people craved the phencyclidine experience, so much so that its use is now believed to have reached epidemic proportions. It is difficult for most observers to understand why this is so. As one researcher said of phencyclidine intoxication, "The hallucinations are usually unpleasant, as indeed is the whole experience resulting from phencyclidine."

As a result of the puzzling increase in the illicit use of PCP, doctors are starting to see many more patients admitted to mental health facilities with PCP psychosis, and phencyclidine-related deaths are being reported with much greater frequency.

Frightening Side Effects

The unpleasant experience of phencyclidine became clear after only a few years' use in surgical practice. It caused frightening hallucinations in as many as 50% of the adults on whom it was used. Even more alarming, it also caused hallucinations in half the children to whom it was given as a surgical anesthetic.

But the hallucinations were only part of the problem. Patients emerging from PCP anesthesia often were in a state of extreme confusion. They had unwelcome, vivid dreams. Sometimes their mental condition was so deranged that doctors used the term emergence psychosis to describe it. This extreme description was justified by the frightening sensations experienced by these unsuspecting patients, sensations that included agitation, anxiety, disorientation, delirium, au-

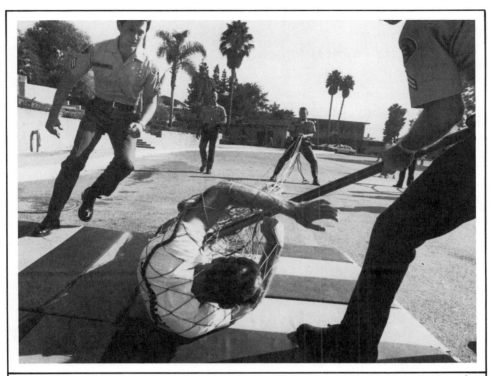

Los Angeles County policemen demonstrate a net used to restrain people who become uncontrollably violent while under the influence of PCP.

ditory hallucinations, and paranoid delusions. Patients found that their thought processes were disordered. In many cases, a state of catatonic stupor developed.

Perhaps most frightening to these people was loss of contact with reality and of the sense of who they were. Many experienced a feeling of depersonalization that was terrifying. Patients described a loss of the ability to distinguish self from nonself, a dissolution of ego boundaries, and a sense of unreality.

Now that many people have illicitly used PCP, their reactions can be compared with those of the surgical patients. Does the experience change when it is expected and even sought after? Apparently not. PCP abusers report the same unpleasant hallucinations, psychoses, thought disorders, and depersonalization that were observed in surgery patients. They also are aware of unpleasant physical sensations that the surgical patients did not experience because they were anesthetized.

PCP and Physical Impairment

Physical effects of PCP include an inability to focus the eyes, walking drunkenly, and muscle rigidity. Loss of voluntary control over the muscles is greatly increased in PCP psychosis, and users can damage their muscles through involuntary muscle contraction.

Physical impairment by PCP is dangerous in its own right. Many people drive while under the influence of PCP. Others try to swim. During one period, two-thirds of the PCP-related deaths in one part of the country were due to drowning.

One of the most frightening aspects of PCP, both to users and to psychiatrists and law-enforcement officials, is the unpredictable nature of the phencyclidine reaction. PCP may unexpectedly bring out aggressive drives in a user. It is associated with violent, homicidal, and suicidal behavior. Perhaps because users feel that they have superhuman strength and invulnerability, more cases of homicide and suicide are associated with PCP than with any other drug of abuse.

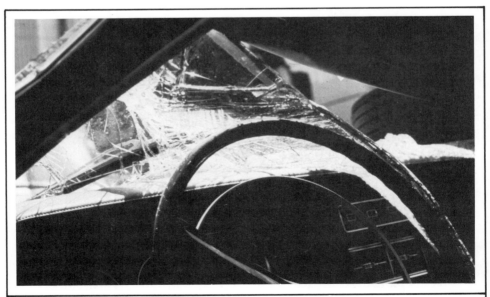

PCP is perhaps the most dangerous and unpredictable of all the psychoactive drugs. Driving under its influence is lethal.

But by far the most damaging effect of phencyclidine is its ability to produce a psychotic state in an individual, as though the drug literally drives a person into a state of madness. If anything, this adverse outcome is more common in voluntary users than it was in surgical patients.

PCP and Mental Illness

PCP is a leading precipitant of psychiatric emergencies. In one study, routine blood samples were taken from 145 consecutive admissions to the Los Angeles County Hospital psychiatric emergency room during a 48-hour period in June 1979. The results showed that 63 samples (more than 40%) were positive for PCP. These patients' symptoms were varied and included mania, depression, and schizophrenia.

The mind-breaking power of phencyclidine was demonstrated dramatically in the fall of 1973 in Washington, D.C. At that time the admission rate for unusually long, severe, and treatment-resistant initial schizophrenic psychoses suddenly tripled in one community mental health center. After some investigation, the doctors realized that they were actually seeing a greatly increased number of cases of PCP psychosis. Phencyclidine's threat to mental stability can be judged from the fact that these psychoses were more severe than true schizophrenia. They were also more severe than cases of LSD psychosis. Mental disorders under LSD last as long as 8 to 16 hours. Some of the cases of PCP psychosis did not resolve for two weeks.

PCP psychosis shares many features with schizophrenia. Both mental states feature hostility, agitation, delusions of grandeur, paranoid delusions, and auditory hallucinations. In PCP psychosis there are also disturbances in thinking — delusional thinking or general intellectual disorganization — that are strikingly reminiscent of the thought disorders seen in schizophrenics.

The sense of depersonalization seen in schizophrenics, that was so alarming to surgery patients anesthetized with phencyclidine is also seen in persons who abuse PCP. There is distortion of the body image, disorientation, and detachment from surroundings. Loss of contact with reality appears to stem from profound disturbance of perceptions. The user loses the ability to integrate sensory input, especially for

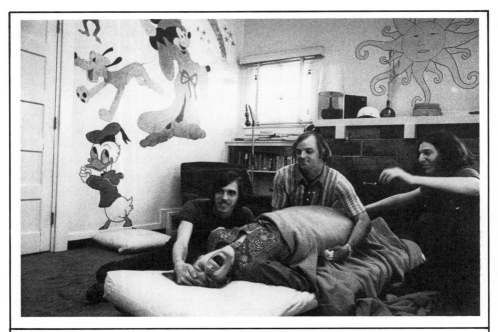

Patients in a drug rehabilitation center demonstrate how to restrain a person who is experiencing a bad trip. Friends cannot manage a bad reaction to PCP, however; it requires immediate medical intervention.

touch and proprioception. Indeed, during testing of the drug before it was approved for human use, investigators observed that subjects entered a state of sensory isolation in which their eyes were wide open but they were unresponsive to the environment.

Some scientists have noted the similarity between this state and the condition of sensory deprivation. They have suggested that PCP induces the characteristics of psychosis by producing sensory deprivation through its far-reaching interference with normal brain chemistry. Certainly sensory deprivation is capable of causing a wide variety of psychotic-like sensations and behaviors, as we saw in Chapter 2.

Even in PCP users who do not suffer acute psychoses, there are fundamental alterations in mental status. For instance, PCP can reactivate latent schizophrenic psychoses or exacerbate schizophrenic symptoms up to several weeks after administration. It causes flashback psychosis even in some individuals who abstain from further PCP consumption following the initial dose. And during periods of abstinence, phencyclidine users may still complain of memory loss, fatigue, irritability, and depression.

One explanation for these problems is that PCP may permanently damage the brain. Indeed, in one study, 6 out of 12 PCP users who had not taken the drug for a long period of time had signs of organic mental impairment.

It is fairly obvious that the risks involved with experimenting with PCP far outweigh any pleasurable feelings it may bring about. For not only does PCP use cause short-term problems such as hallucinations and various other perceptual distortions, its effects can become long-term, with flashbacks taking place years after the last time the drug was taken. But far more serious than this is the risk PCP presents to even its most casual, first-time user; that is, the risk of severe and irreversible perceptual distortions and mental illness.

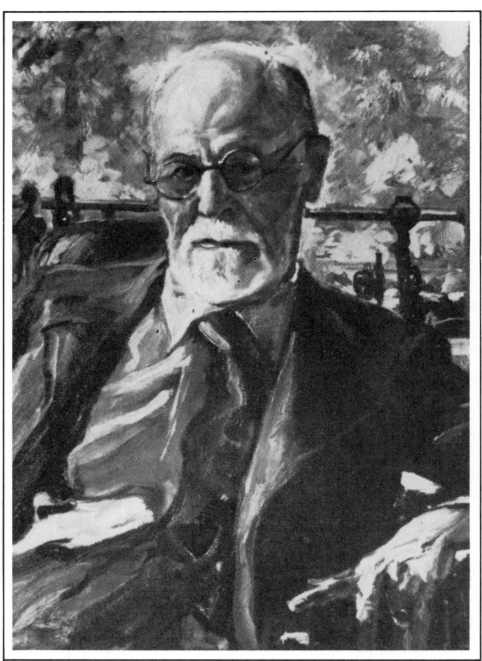

Sigmund Freud, the founder of psychoanalysis. Although he would later change his mind, Freud was for a time an advocate of cocaine use, claiming that it induced "lasting euphoria."

CHAPTER 7

COCAINE AND INHALANTS

Although hallucinogens and opiates are the drugs that are most popularly believed to affect perceptions, various other drugs cause their share of distortions, as well. Drugs such as cocaine and inhalants all have dangerous side effects, severe perceptual disturbances among them. Repeated cocaine use can result in a loss of the sense of self; experimentation with inhalants often induces vivid hallucinations. These disruptions of the normal mind are no less disturbing or even, in some cases, life threatening, than those brought on by the use of heroin or LSD.

Cocaine

It gave me a sense of well-being, like I was worth something.
—former high-dose cocaine user

In previous chapters we have covered several drugs that alter the user's perceptions of the external world. With cocaine, however, we come to a unique chemical entity. Cocaine is unlike any of the previous illicit drugs we have discussed in several ways. Its pharmacology — how it produces its psychological and perceptual effects — is unique. Its addictive potential is dramatic and may even be greater than that of heroin. Some experts believe that susceptible individuals can become dependent on cocaine with a single use.

One possible contributing factor is that cocaine can be taken in many forms — powder, freebase, crack — and by many routes. Cocaine's ability to entrap its victims is also greater because of its acceptance by certain segments of middle-class and professional America, perhaps because it does not require a needle for injection and so has escaped the stigma of the primarily lower-class narcotic heroin.

But probably the most dangerous of the many unique aspects of cocaine is the type of illusion it creates in the user. Cocaine does not create an alteration of sensory perception. Rather, it produces major distortions of the sense of self, the most basic perceptions of a person's own character and personality.

Lester Grinspoon and James Bakalar, in their classic 1976 book *Cocaine: A Drug and Its Social Evolution*, differentiate cocaine from opiates such as heroin:

> Opiates tend to cause a loss of interest in the self that makes mastery of the external environment irrelevant; the feeling is a kind of nirvana. In contrast, a stimulant like cocaine heightens the sensory and emotional brightness and distinctiveness of the self against its environmental background.

The tricks cocaine plays on the mind were summed up by one researcher in the phrase "an illusory satisfaction of desires." The desires to which he refers are the unmet psychological needs of the immature ego. One physician who has treated many patients for cocaine overdose calls a chronic experienced cocaine user "one who has dwelt upon the psychic summit of the premier ego-enhancing drug."

Although he later reversed himself, the Viennese physician and founder of psychoanalysis, Sigmund Freud, was for a time an advocate of cocaine. He wrote:

> The psychic effect of [cocaine] in doses of [50–100 mg] consists of exhilaration and lasting euphoria, which does not differ in any way from the normal euphoria of a healthy person. . . . One is simply normal, and soon finds it difficult to believe that one is under the influence of any drug at all.

As we shall see, cocaine does stimulate the central nervous system. But the price paid for this stimulation is exorbitant. Cocaine both deludes the mind into perceiving the self as a

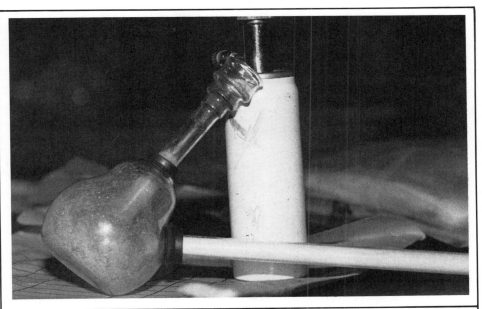

A pipe used for smoking crack, an extremely addictive form of cocaine. Crack use has recently reached epidemic proportions.

god and stimulates the body to such a high level that it soon wears out and loses the ability to function without the artifical urgings of the drug.

Effects on the Nervous System

Pharmacologically, cocaine exerts a very strong stimulant effect on both the brain and the peripheral nerves. That puts it in the same category as amphetamines. But cocaine is a stronger stimulant than amphetamines, and the high it produces is more transient and more subtle (at least in smaller doses when taken by nose).

Cocaine has many effects on the nervous system that become apparent a short time after administration. These include the following:

- euphoria, nonstop talking, restlessness, excitement
- an increase in perceptual awareness and cognitive speed
- an increased capacity for muscular work (lessened sense of fatigue)
- restlessness, irritability and apprehension, pacing

The state of high stimulation found in cocaine users has been described as "armed," taken from the word "armado" used by Peruvian natives who chew coca leaves. It is a state of hyperalertness. "Any rapid or unexpected movement on the part of those around him may be interpreted as hostile," warns one doctor who has treated many persons for toxic cocaine reactions.

Psychological Effects

The physical excitement produced by cocaine is paralleled by an equal psychological excitement. Cocaine produces a strong state of psychological excitation involving feelings of euphoria more pronounced than those seen with practically any other psychoactive agent, including heroin. Psychological depression, however, follows this state in a rather short time (30 minutes).

Says one researcher: "One of the qualities of a cocaine high is that, initially, it makes you feel powerful and in control. Of course, this feeling is short-lived (two to 40 minutes, depending upon dose and quality), and the crash back to reality can be rather harsh; but abusers and addicts largely ignore all negative aspects and keep going for that increasingly illusory sense of well-being."

Users have described cocaine's seductive psychological effects in various words:

- "king of the mountain, on top of the world; powerful and in control"

- "like you can accomplish whatever you want"

- "even if you are inadequate and painfully shy, it makes you feel better about yourself; it gives you the courage to socialize"

- "the greatest ego-inflating drug there is"

An extreme example of the alteration in self-image produced by cocaine was presented by a researcher who in 1926 convinced several of his fellow physicians to volunteer for injections of cocaine under the skin. Offerman reported that one woman doctor "felt coquettish and turned her eyes with enlarged pupils on the experimenter, wanted to dance, and regarded her own behavior as affected and slightly ridiculous."

The aftereffect of the cocaine high — the price to be paid for feeling godlike — is often a personal hell. One aspect of this hell is cocaine paranoia, as described by Grinspoon and Bakalar:

> This strong focal awareness [on the self] may degenerate into a paranoia. Everything and everbody seem to be threatening "me," the object of greatest interest in the universe.

Other consequences of chronic high-dose use include the following:

- nervousness and unrelieved fatigue

- lapses in attention, inability to concentrate, situational sexual impotency; pseudohallucinations: illusions that the user perceives but recognizes as unreal

- tactile hallucinations, particularly "cocaine bugs" in the skin

- visual hallucinations, called "snow lights"

- auditory hallucinations, the feeling that "footsteps are following me"

- severe depression when not "wired"

Frequent users may become so psychologically excited and agitated that they develop an intense anxiety state with paranoid features. In this state, hallucinations are not uncommon, and abnormal sensations induced by cocaine in the peripheral nerves may convince the hyperexcited user that animals are burrowing under his skin. These are the so-called cocaine bugs. One actress required plastic surgery after clawing her face open in response to these tactile illusions.

Cocaine is not addictive in the same sense as heroin; that is, no clear withdrawal symptoms are seen upon discontinuing use of the drug. But it does induce a very powerful psychological dependence in susceptible persons. Explains one physician who treats cocaine users:

> For some individuals who feel profoundly oppressed by a cruel, capricious, and overwhelming world, cocaine can, however fleetingly, make the unbearable seem bearable. These properties can lead to the highest degree of psychic dependence.

This dependence can be heard in the voice of this former cocaine user:

> I lost job after job and I couldn't work and we were on assistance. Oh yeah, I die for it every time I think of it. But it does me absolutely no good. I get terrible hallucinations. I get the horrors something awful. . . . I get as paranoid as you could possibly get. . . . I see secret tunnels opening in the walls. And yet, if by some mischance they started to give it to me, I wouldn't refuse it. I would try to rationalize it . . . that I would manage it better this time. But I wouldn't.

Cocaine addicts even have difficulty admitting that the drug is bad for them. They cannot face giving it up, cannot face the fact that something that makes them feel so good could be so destructive. Reluctance to face the destruction of his life is clear in this exchange between a user and a therapist who is helping him quit:

> *Therapist*: It must have been pretty lonely sitting in your study, by yourself, locking your wife out of your life, and snorting cocaine all through the night.
> *Jed*: I'm not sure I'm convinced yet, but I can see how important cocaine has become. It's true. I did lock my wife out of my life, and she has always been very important to me. No wonder she thought I might have a mistress. I did, only her name was cocaine.

Glue Sniffing

"Glue sniffing" refers to more than getting high by inhaling glue. It is a general term applied to the abuse of any substance that easily forms a vapor under normal conditions. Substances that release vapors are called volatile chemicals, or inhalants. Most of the inhalants that are sniffed for their mind-altering properties are hydrocarbons (molecules composed of carbon and hydrogen) and, sometimes, oxygen.

Sniffing inhalants for their psychoactive effects became popular in the mid-1970s as an activity almost restricted to teenagers. In 1983, it was estimated that 1 in 10 people under the age of 17 had experimented with inhalants at some time.

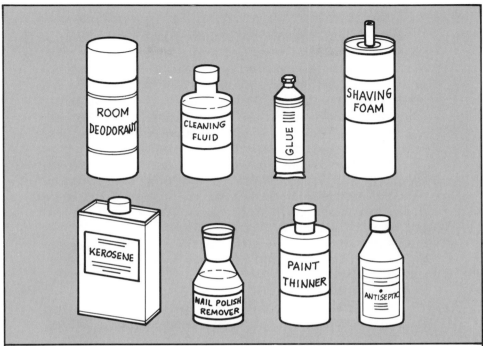

An artist's rendering of various substances whose fumes are sniffed for their intoxicating properties. This potentially lethal form of substance abuse is almost exclusively restricted to teenagers.

The reason for this and for the almost exclusive use of inhalants by teenagers is probably that inhalants are both legal and easily located and obtained. In addition to the model or airplane glue that is most often favored (for its organic solvent, toluene), such organic chemicals as benzene (used for cleaning spots from clothes), paint thinner, nail-polish remover, kerosene, and gasoline are frequently used.

Another class of volatile hydrocarbons that are inhaled are fluorocarbons, volatile hydrocarbons that contain a fluorine atom. These were used as propellants in aerosol cans before concern for their effect on the atmosphere caused them to be banned. Some common products dispensed in aerosol cans by means of fluorocarbons include whipped cream, shaving cream, antiseptics, hair spray, and room deodorizers. Today, some fluorocarbons such as Freon, which is used as a coolant in refrigerators and air conditioners, are still available.

Side Effects of Inhalant Abuse

Inhaling volatile hydrocarbons alters perceptions in many vivid ways, in a sense putting it in the same league as marijuana and other psychedelic drugs. But there are two important facts about glue sniffing that set it apart from the other psychoactive drugs. First, unlike any other drug abuse, it is practiced almost exclusively by young people. Second, it carries a greater risk of causing sudden death than any other substance we have discussed.

Physically, the sensory effects of volatile fluorocarbons, especially toluene, are similar to those of alcohol, as is the biologic mechanism by which the two substances achieve their effects. Both volatile fluorocarbons and alcohol are central nervous system depressants as well as sedatives. This means that they both lower the activity of certain groups of brain cells that raise conscious barriers to certain feelings and actions, which explains how these drugs produce bizarre and unusual behavior.

Volatile fluorocarbons, however, are much stronger than the usual concentrations of alcohol consumed in social set-

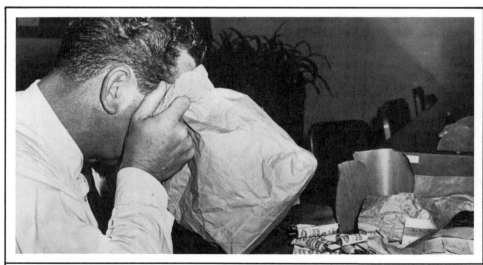

A 1962 photograph shows a law enforcement official demonstrating one method of sniffing glue. Sniffing glue carries more risk of sudden death than the use of any other known psychoactive substance.

tings. They are also more unpredictable and have far more unpleasant side effects. Whereas an alcohol binge may leave the drinker sleepy or with a headache, glue sniffing might give him vivid nightmares.

Of course, a drug must have some desirable effect to be used by so many people, and inhalants are no exception. Glue sniffing produces a sense of excitement and euphoria in its users, but these effects are illusory and temporary at best. For upon the heels of the pleasant feelings comes a much darker side to these drugs.

One of the first and most prominent effects of glue sniffing is a loud buzzing noise that has no apparent origin and is typically perceived as disorienting. The sense of solidity and weight that we find so comforting can also be lost after an episode of glue sniffing, leaving the user with a feeling of lightness or a floating sensation. One user related that she felt "an urge to want to walk out a window."

Illusions, usually manifested in visual hallucinations, are another common side effect of inhalant intoxication. Very often a red light is a prominent feature of these imaginary scenes. Typical descriptions of illusions by teenagers who abused inhalants include "little red and green men darting about like fireflies" and "bright lights flaring."

In the early phase of an episode induced by volatile substances, most users perceive these illusions as pleasant and entertaining. After a period of time, however, the drug state changes character, and fearful images predominate. As one authority in the field reported: "Delusions of perception gradually give way to hallucinations followed by stupor and unconsciousness." One girl related this description of a frightening illusion that combined distortions of sight, hearing, and touch:

> Everything went dark and there was red light everywhere. Insects and horrible crawly things were all around and I could hear monsters moaning and coming nearer. Something with a horrible face got hold of my neck and I was so scared I just screamed and screamed.

This description is comparable to the frightening hallucinations produced by long-term severe abuse of alcohol, called *delirium tremens*, or the DT's.

Another girl who sniffed volatile solvents suffered a frightening experience that was similar to delirium tremens in a different way, the feeling of repulsive creatures crawling on her skin. She was discovered, still intoxicated by the solvent, repeatedly crying out, "Get off me," while staring wild-eyed at the floors and walls of the room and acting terrified. This episode was quite real and frightening for her, and one year later she still feared even talking about it.

In the early phase of solvent inhalant abuse, these long-lasting effects are not quite so common. For the most part, the perceptual distortions fade as the drug wears off. But habitual glue sniffing initiates a series of more permanent sensory disturbances. These are accompanied by psychological changes such as confusion, disorientation, and loss of self-control. With further use, the person loses basic contact with reality and begins to perceive life as a dream state.

Ultimately, with habitual use, more startling changes take place. In the last stage of volatile hydrocarbon intoxication, perception remains disturbed even after the last dose of the drug has worn off. The extent and variety of these distortions are great, as well.

Sensory perception becomes grossly and permanently distorted. Users may feel as though unseen hands are being run over their bodies or that their skin is being pricked with needles. The toes and fingers may become numb for no physical reason. Noise may become a very offensive sensation, with sounds becoming disturbingly loud. Vision can become defective, the ability to focus may be altered, or double-vision may appear. Users may also smell familiar things even when they are not present.

In addition to the distorted sensations, auditory or visual hallucinations usually take place. A user may start hearing voices or have conversations with God or the devil, just as people suffering from schizophrenia do. Sometimes visions of monsters will appear. One 15-year-old girl reported seeing illusions of Dracula coming through the wall to get her:

He was horrible, blood dripping from his mouth. People were lying dead on the floor. I went to see my brother and he was just a skeleton lying on the bed. I ran in to see my two sisters who were just skeletons. I was terrified!

Internal proprioceptive sensations are also disturbed. There may be pain in various parts of the body — the legs, side, or stomach. The individual may become acutely aware of his heartbeat and experience palpitations. The sense of balance is often disturbed, creating the sensation that the ground is moving.

Perceptions of the self, too, are typically disoriented. For instance, users may begin to feel that they are not real or that the self is not really present. They may begin to look at themselves from the outside. With still other users, the opposite sets in. Their sense of power may be augmented, cre-

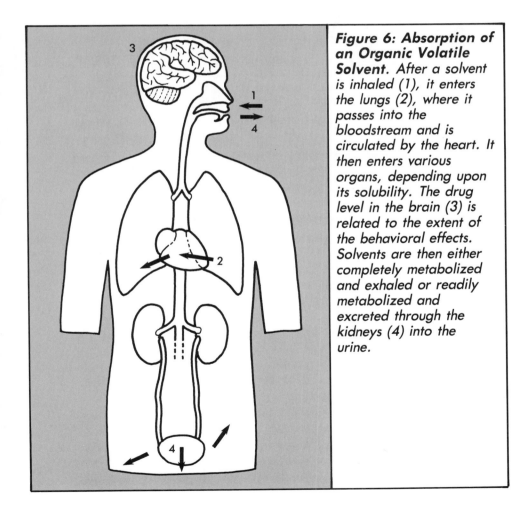

Figure 6: Absorption of an Organic Volatile Solvent. *After a solvent is inhaled (1), it enters the lungs (2), where it passes into the bloodstream and is circulated by the heart. It then enters various organs, depending upon its solubility. The drug level in the brain (3) is related to the extent of the behavioral effects. Solvents are then either completely metabolized and exhaled or readily metabolized and excreted through the kidneys (4) into the urine.*

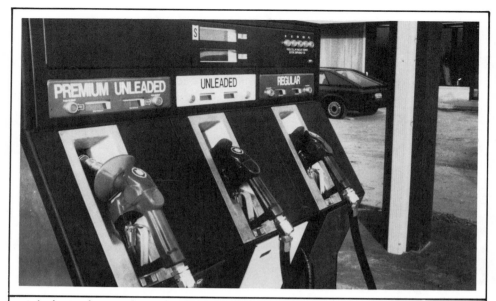

Inhalant abusers have been known to sniff gasoline fumes in search of a high. The effects of inhalants on mood and perception result from their destructive actions on the central nervous system.

ating the feeling of being able to fly or perform superhuman feats. A sense of confusion can also set in, leading to groundless fears, in conjunction with paranoia and suicidal thoughts.

What is, in reality, being experienced is the destructive effect of the inhalants on the nervous system. Beyond the ears, eyes, nose, and skin, along the nerves, vapors are eating away at vital parts of the nervous system, damaging its ability to function normally. Nerves begin to short-circuit or to fire off messages spontaneously, without waiting for signals from the sense organs.

The Ultimate Bad Trip

Just one dose of an inhalant can be fatal. There have been many recorded instances of teenagers dying a horrible death after inhaling a volatile chemical. These deaths are not due to an overdose, however, but rather to an unexpected and unpredictable reaction to the chemicals. This sudden death can result at any time, in any instance, regardless of whether the person has used the same drug before. Aerosol sprays, which contain fluorocarbons, have been particularly linked to heart failure and death.

In one case, a group of teenagers were sniffing from an aerosol spray. They had sniffed glue before with no problems. Suddenly, one boy began gasping and running wildly. After he had gone a short distance, he staggered and fell. When the rest of the group, including his younger brother, caught up to him, they saw that he was suffocating before their very eyes. An ambulance came, but it was too late. The boy had had a toxic reaction to the fluorocarbon contained in the spray can, and his heart had stopped beating.

The above experience points out the depth of the risks involved in glue sniffing. Young people who engage in this activity are usually unaware that it can kill them at any time. And if they are not killed but continue to use inhalants, they leave themselves open to permanent sensory damage.

Conclusion

The perceptual distortions caused by the drugs discussed in this volume can range from mild to severe, from transitory to permanent. The longer a psychoactive drug is used, the more destructive its effects are likely to be. However, there really is no predicting what consequences drug use will have on any given user at any given time, whether he or she is experimenting with an illicit substance for the first time or using it habitually. To be sure, psychoactive drugs can in fact create heightened sensory experiences; indeed, this is a great part of their allure. In the final analysis, though, derangement of the senses is a classic characteristic of madness, and no drug experience is worth the risk.

APPENDIX

State Agencies
for the Prevention and Treatment
of Drug Abuse

ALABAMA
Department of Mental Health
Division of Mental Illness and
  Substance Abuse Community
  Programs
200 Interstate Park Drive
P.O. Box 3710
Montgomery, AL 36193
(205) 271-9253

ALASKA
Department of Health and Social
  Services
Office of Alcoholism and Drug
  Abuse
Pouch H-05-F
Juneau, AK 99811
(907) 586-6201

ARIZONA
Department of Health Services
Division of Behavioral Health
  Services
Bureau of Community Services
Alcohol Abuse and Alcoholism
  Section
2500 East Van Buren
Phoenix, AZ 85008
(602) 255-1238

Department of Health Services
Division of Behavioral Health
  Services
Bureau of Community Services
Drug Abuse Section
2500 East Van Buren
Phoenix, AZ 85008
(602) 255-1240

ARKANSAS
Department of Human Services
Office of Alcohol and Drug Abuse
  Prevention
1515 West 7th Avenue
Suite 310
Little Rock, AR 72202
(501) 371-2603

CALIFORNIA
Department of Alcohol and Drug
  Abuse
111 Capitol Mall
Sacramento, CA 95814
(916) 445-1940

COLORADO
Department of Health
Alcohol and Drug Abuse Division
4210 East 11th Avenue
Denver, CO 80220
(303) 320-6137

CONNECTICUT
Alcohol and Drug Abuse
  Commission
999 Asylum Avenue
3rd Floor
Hartford, CT 06105
(203) 566-4145

DELAWARE
Division of Mental Health
Bureau of Alcoholism and Drug
  Abuse
1901 North Dupont Highway
Newcastle, DE 19720
(302) 421-6101

DISTRICT OF COLUMBIA
Department of Human Services
Office of Health Planning and
  Development
601 Indiana Avenue, NW
Suite 500
Washington, D.C. 20004
(202) 724-5641

FLORIDA
Department of Health and
  Rehabilitative Services
Alcoholic Rehabilitation Program
1317 Winewood Boulevard
Room 187A
Tallahassee, FL 32301
(904) 488-0396

Department of Health and
  Rehabilitative Services
Drug Abuse Program
1317 Winewood Boulevard
Building 6, Room 155
Tallahassee, FL 32301
(904) 488-0900

GEORGIA
Department of Human Resources
Division of Mental Health and
  Mental Retardation
Alcohol and Drug Section
618 Ponce De Leon Avenue, NE
Atlanta, GA 30365-2101
(404) 894-4785

HAWAII
Department of Health
Mental Health Division
Alcohol and Drug Abuse Branch
1250 Punch Bowl Street
P.O. Box 3378
Honolulu, HI 96801
(808) 548-4280

IDAHO
Department of Health and Welfare
Bureau of Preventive Medicine
Substance Abuse Section
450 West State
Boise, ID 83720
(208) 334-4368

ILLINOIS
Department of Mental Health and
  Developmental Disabilities
Division of Alcoholism
160 North La Salle Street
Room 1500
Chicago, IL 60601
(312) 793-2907

Illinois Dangerous Drugs
  Commission
300 North State Street
Suite 1500
Chicago, IL 60610
(312) 822-9860

INDIANA
Department of Mental Health
Division of Addiction Services
429 North Pennsylvania Street
Indianapolis, IN 46204
(317) 232-7816

IOWA
Department of Substance Abuse
505 5th Avenue
Insurance Exchange Building
Suite 202
Des Moines, IA 50319
(515) 281-3641

KANSAS
Department of Social Rehabilitation
Alcohol and Drug Abuse Services
2700 West 6th Street
Biddle Building
Topeka, KS 66606
(913) 296-3925

KENTUCKY
Cabinet for Human Resources
Department of Health Services
Substance Abuse Branch
275 East Main Street
Frankfort, KY 40601
(502) 564-2880

LOUISIANA
Department of Health and Human
  Resources
Office of Mental Health and
  Substance Abuse
655 North 5th Street
P.O. Box 4049
Baton Rouge, LA 70821
(504) 342-2565

MAINE
Department of Human Services
Office of Alcoholism and Drug
  Abuse Prevention
Bureau of Rehabilitation
32 Winthrop Street
Augusta, ME 04330
(207) 289-2781

MARYLAND
Alcoholism Control Administration
201 West Preston Street
Fourth Floor
Baltimore, MD 21201
(301) 383-2977

State Health Department
Drug Abuse Administration
201 West Preston Street
Baltimore, MD 21201
(301) 383-3312

MASSACHUSETTS
Department of Public Health
Division of Alcoholism
755 Boylston Street
Sixth Floor
Boston, MA 02116
(617) 727-1960

Department of Public Health
Division of Drug Rehabilitation
600 Washington Street
Boston, MA 02114
(617) 727-8617

MICHIGAN
Department of Public Health
Office of Substance Abuse Services
3500 North Logan Street
P.O. Box 30035
Lansing, MI 48909
(517) 373-8603

MINNESOTA
Department of Public Welfare
Chemical Dependency Program
  Division
Centennial Building
658 Cedar Street
4th Floor
Saint Paul, MN 55155
(612) 296-4614

MISSISSIPPI
Department of Mental Health
Division of Alcohol and Drug Abuse
1102 Robert E. Lee Building
Jackson, MS 39201
(601) 359-1297

MISSOURI
Department of Mental Health
Division of Alcoholism and Drug
  Abuse
2002 Missouri Boulevard
P.O. Box 687
Jefferson City, MO 65102
(314) 751-4942

MONTANA
Department of Institutions
Alcohol and Drug Abuse Division
1539 11th Avenue
Helena, MT 59620
(406) 449-2827

NEBRASKA
Department of Public Institutions
Division of Alcoholism and Drug
Abuse
801 West Van Dorn Street
P.O. Box 94728
Lincoln, NB 68509
(402) 471-2851, Ext. 415

NEVADA
Department of Human Resources
Bureau of Alcohol and Drug Abuse
505 East King Street
Carson City, NV 89710
(702) 885-4790

NEW HAMPSHIRE
Department of Health and Welfare
Office of Alcohol and Drug Abuse
   Prevention
Hazen Drive
Health and Welfare Building
Concord, NH 03301
(603) 271-4627

NEW JERSEY
Department of Health
Division of Alcoholism
129 East Hanover Street CN 362
Trenton, NJ 08625
(609) 292-8949

Department of Health
Division of Narcotic and Drug
   Abuse Control
129 East Hanover Street CN 362
Trenton, NJ 08625
(609) 292-8949

NEW MEXICO
Health and Environment Department
Behavioral Services Division
Substance Abuse Bureau
725 Saint Michaels Drive
P.O. Box 968
Santa Fe, NM 87503
(505) 984-0020, Ext. 304

NEW YORK
Division of Alcoholism and Alcohol
   Abuse
194 Washington Avenue
Albany, NY 12210
(518) 474-5417

Division of Substance Abuse
   Services
Executive Park South
Box 8200
Albany, NY 12203
(518) 457-7629

NORTH CAROLINA
Department of Human Resources
Division of Mental Health, Mental
   Retardation and Substance Abuse
   Services
Alcohol and Drug Abuse Services
325 North Salisbury Street
Albemarle Building
Raleigh, NC 27611
(919) 733-4670

NORTH DAKOTA
Department of Human Services
Division of Alcoholism and Drug
   Abuse
State Capitol Building
Bismarck, ND 58505
(701) 224-2767

OHIO
Department of Health
Division of Alcoholism
246 North High Street
P.O. Box 118
Columbus, OH 43216
(614) 466-3543

Department of Mental Health
Bureau of Drug Abuse
65 South Front Street
Columbus, OH 43215
(614) 466-9023

OKLAHOMA
Department of Mental Health
Alcohol and Drug Programs
4545 North Lincoln Boulevard
Suite 100 East Terrace
P.O. Box 53277
Oklahoma City, OK 73152
(405) 521-0044

OREGON
Department of Human Resources
Mental Health Division
Office of Programs for Alcohol and
    Drug Problems
2575 Bittern Street, NE
Salem, OR 97310
(503) 378-2163

PENNSYLVANIA
Department of Health
Office of Drug and Alcohol
    Programs
Commonwealth and Forster Avenues
Health and Welfare Building
P.O. Box 90
Harrisburg, PA 17108
(717) 787-9857

RHODE ISLAND
Department of Mental Health,
    Mental Retardation and Hospitals
Division of Substance Abuse
Substance Abuse Administration
    Building
Cranston, RI 02920
(401) 464-2091

SOUTH CAROLINA
Commission on Alcohol and Drug
    Abuse
3700 Forest Drive
Columbia, SC 29204
(803) 758-2521

SOUTH DAKOTA
Department of Health
Division of Alcohol and Drug Abuse
523 East Capitol, Joe Foss Building
Pierre, SD 57501
(605) 773-4806

TENNESSEE
Department of Mental Health and
    Mental Retardation
Alcohol and Drug Abuse Services
505 Deaderick Street
James K. Polk Building,
    Fourth Floor
Nashville, TN 37219
(615) 741-1921

TEXAS
Commission on Alcoholism
809 Sam Houston State Office
    Building
Austin, TX 78701
(512) 475-2577
Department of Community Affairs
Drug Abuse Prevention Division
2015 South Interstate Highway 35
P.O. Box 13166
Austin, TX 78711
(512) 443-4100

UTAH
Department of Social Services
Division of Alcoholism and Drugs
150 West North Temple
Suite 350
P.O. Box 2500
Salt Lake City, UT 84110
(801) 533-6532

VERMONT
Agency of Human Services
Department of Social and
    Rehabilitation Services
Alcohol and Drug Abuse Division
103 South Main Street
Waterbury, VT 05676
(802) 241-2170

VIRGINIA
Department of Mental Health and
   Mental Retardation
Division of Substance Abuse
109 Governor Street
P.O. Box 1797
Richmond, VA 23214
(804) 786-5313

WASHINGTON
Department of Social and Health
   Service
Bureau of Alcohol and Substance
   Abuse
Office Building—44 W
Olympia, WA 98504
(206) 753-5866

WEST VIRGINIA
Department of Health
Office of Behavioral Health Services
Division on Alcoholism and Drug
   Abuse
1800 Washington Street East
Building 3 Room 451
Charleston, WV 25305
(304) 348-2276

WISCONSIN
Department of Health and Social
   Services
Division of Community Services
Bureau of Community Programs
Alcohol and Other Drug Abuse
   Program Office
1 West Wilson Street
P.O. Box 7851
Madison, WI 53707
(608) 266-2717

WYOMING
Alcohol and Drug Abuse Programs
Hathaway Building
Cheyenne, WY 82002
(307) 777-7115, Ext. 7118

GUAM
Mental Health & Substance Abuse
   Agency
P.O. Box 20999
Guam 96921

PUERTO RICO
Department of Addiction Control
   Services
Alcohol Abuse Programs
P.O. Box B-Y Rio Piedras Station
Rio Piedras, PR 00928
(809) 763-5014

Department of Addiction Control
   Services
Drug Abuse Programs
P.O. Box B-Y Rio Piedras Station
Rio Piedras, PR 00928
(809) 764-8140

VIRGIN ISLANDS
Division of Mental Health,
   Alcoholism & Drug Dependency
   Services
P.O. Box 7329
Saint Thomas, Virgin Islands 00801
(809) 774-7265

AMERICAN SAMOA
LBJ Tropical Medical Center
Department of Mental Health Clinic
Pago Pago, American Samoa 96799

TRUST TERRITORIES
Director of Health Services
Office of the High Commissioner
Saipan, Trust Territories 96950

Further Reading

Baum, Joanne. *One Step Over the Line*. San Francisco: Harper & Row, 1985.

Blum, Richard H. *Utopiates: The Use & Users of LSD 25*. New York: Atherton Press, 1964.

Brimblecombe, Roger W., and Roger M. Pinder. *Hallucinogenic Agents*. Bristol, England: Wright-Scientechnica, 1975.

Carso, John F. *The Experimental Psychology of Sensory Behavior*. New York: Holt, Rinehart & Winston, 1967.

Cornacchia, Harold J., David J. Bentel, and David E. Smith. *Drugs in the Classroom*. St. Louis, MO: Mosby, 1973.

Grinspoon, Lester. *Marihuana Reconsidered*. Cambridge: Harvard University Press, 1971.

Grinspoon, Lester, and James B. Bakalar. *Cocaine: A Drug & Its Social Evolution*. New York: Basic Books, 1976.

Jacobs, Barry L. *Hallucinogens: Neurochemical, Behavioral, and Clinical Perspectives*. New York: Dodd, Mead, 1985.

Miller, Loren L. *Marijuana: Effects on Human Behavior*. New York: Academic Press, 1974.

Moreau, Jacques-Joseph. *Hashish and Mental Illness*. New York: Raven Press, 1973.

O'Connor, Denis. *Glue Sniffing and Volatile Substance Abuse*. Aldershot, England: Gower, 1983.

Stimson, G. V. *Heroin and Behavior: Diversity Among Addicts Attending London Clinics*. New York: Wiley, 1973.

Glossary

acute toxic psychosis a "bad trip"; an adverse reaction to the LSD experience due to its effect on the central nervous system; includes acute paranoia, grandiose or persecutory illusions, and a panic reaction

addiction a condition caused by repeated drug use, characterized by a compulsive urge to continue using the drug, a tendency to increase the dosage, and physiological and/or psychological dependence

amphetamine any one of a number of drugs that act to stimulate parts of the central nervous system

anticholinergics natural compounds found in henbane, belladonna, and mandrake, which produce disturbing hallucinations, a state of confusion, agitation, and a loss of memory

belladonna the deadly nightshade plant, parts of which are used as a narcotic and to dilate the pupils

cholinergic system a chemical system of the brain

cocaine the primary psychoactive ingredient in the coca plant; functions as a behavioral stimulant

cochlea a spiral tube of the inner ear resembling a snail shell and having nerve endings necessary for hearing

delirium tremens also known as $\widehat{DT}$'s; a condition caused by abrupt withdrawal of alcohol or sedatives when the patient is addicted to the drug; characterized by violent trembling and hallucinations

depressant a drug that depresses the central nervous system; used to help people block out unpleasant thoughts and anxieties and reduce tensions

dimethyltryptamine also known as DMT; a powerful psychedelic drug prepared from the beans of the South American *Piptadenia peregrina* tree

ergot alkaloids a group of chemicals made by the fungus *Claviceps purpurea*, which grows on rye and other grains

ergotism a disease condition produced in humans who eat flour made from grain affected by the various fungi of the genus *Claviceps*

flashbacks the return of hallucinogenic images after the immediate effects of hallucinogens have worn off; including perceptual distortions, heightened imagery, and recurrent images

hallucination a sensory impression that has no basis in reality

heroin a semisynthetic opiate produced by a chemical modification of morphine

inhalant any substance that easily forms a vapor under normal conditions

kinesthesia a proprioceptive sensation that tells what the body is doing to create motion, where body parts are, and how they are moving

lysergic acid diethylamide LSD; a hallucinogenic drug derived from a fungus that grows on rye or from morning-glory seeds

mandragora officinarum mandrake; a plant that is a natural hallucinogen bearing purplish flowers and having a branched root, thought to look like a human body

mescaline a psychedelic drug found in the peyote cactus

narcotic originally referring to a group of drugs producing similar effects to those of morphine; often used to refer to any substance that sedates, has a depressive effect, or causes dependence

opiate any compound from the milky juice of the poppy plant *Papaver somniferum* including opium, morphine, codeine, and heroin

paranoid schizophrenia psychosis a psychiatric disorder characterized by extreme suspicion and an altered view of reality

perception a mental impression received through the sense organs and produced by the brain

peyote an organic hallucinatory drug used usually for medicinal and ceremonial purposes by some American Indians

phencyclidine PCP; also known as angel dust; a potent preparation that is mixed with other drugs to enhance their side effects, it can produce dangerous and terrifying hallucinations or psychotic reactions

physical dependence an adaption of the body to the presence of a drug such that its absence produces withdrawal symptoms

proprioceptive sense a sense that receives and interprets signals from inside the body to determine the relation of the internal to the external world; balance is a proprioceptive sense

psilocybin a strongly hallucinogenic compound derived from the mushroom *Psilocybe mexicana*

psychedelic producing hallucinations or having mind-altering properties

psychological dependence a condition in which the user craves a drug to maintain a sense of well-being and feels discomfort when deprived of it

psychotomimetic any drug that induces psychotic symptoms

receptor a specialized component of a cell that combines with a chemical substance to alter the function of a cell; nerve cell receptors combine with neurotransmitters

retina a delicate light-sensitive membrane lining the inner eyeball and connected to the brain by the optic nerve

schizophrenia a mental disorder in which a person loses touch with reality; characterized by a profound emotional withdrawal and bizarre behavior, often includes delusions and hallucinations

tolerance a decrease of susceptibility to the effects of a drug due to its continued administration, resulting in the user's need to increase the drug dosage in order to achieve the effects experienced previously

tympanic membrane the thin semitransparent membrane separating the middle and the external ear

vertigo the sensation of dizziness

withdrawal the psychological and physiological effects of the discontinued use of a drug

PICTURE CREDITS

Index

hearing
  hallucinations and, 33
  mechanism, 26–27
Heffter, A., 57
henbane, 55–56, 77. *See also*
    hallucinogens
heroin, 71, 73–74, 85–86. *See also*
    opiates
Hofmann, Albert, 54–55, 58–60, 63. *See
    also* LSD
Hollister, Leo, 55
Huxley, Aldous, 62
hydrocarbons, 90, 94. *See also* inhalants
hyoscine, 55. *See also* hallucinogens
Hyoscyamus niger, 55
hypnosis, 69

inhalants
  aftereffects, 96–97
  deaths from, 96–97
  epidemiology, 90, 92
  hallucinations and, 93–94
  mechanism of action, 92–93
  perceptual effects, 93–96
  psychological effects, 95–96
  reasons for use, 90–91
  risks, 92
  types, 90–91

James, William, 57
jimson weed, 55, 77. *See also*
    hallucinogens

kinesthesia, 35
Kluver, Heinrich, 57

Lewin, Louis, 61
locoweed, 55. *See also* hallucinogens
LSD (lysergic acid diethylamide), 20, 69,
    77–78, 85. *See also*
    hallucinogens
  aftereffects, 66–67
  chemistry, 54, 60
  discovery, 55, 58–59
  flashbacks, 24, 60, 63–65
  hallucinogenic effects, 56, 59, 62–63
  mechanism of action, 60–61
  "peak experiences" and, 65–66
  perceptual changes, 62–63, 66
  potency, 57, 59–60
  religion and, 66–67
  risks, 24, 60, 63–65, 67
lysergic acid diethylamide. *See* LSD

Mandragora officinalis, 55
mandrake, 55–56. *See also* hallucinogens
mania, 81
marijuana, 20, 35. *See also* THC
  cognitive effects, 49–51
  coordination and, 40–41, 47–48
  driving and, 47–48
  interaction with LSD, 64
  memory and, 40–41, 49–51
  methods of studying effects, 39
  music and, 43–44
  perceptual effects, 40–45
  psychoactive effects, 40–43
  risks, 40, 47–48, 50–51
  sexuality and, 48–49
  space perception and, 47
  time perception and, 44–46
Maslow, Abraham, 65–66
mescaline, 54, 56–57, 60–61, 69, 78. *See
    also* hallucinogens
methamphetamine, 36
methaqualone. *See* Quaalude
morphine, 71. *See also* opiates
muscimol, 55. *See also* hallucinogens
Mysteries of Eleusis, 60

narcotics, 69–71. *See also* opiates
National Institutes of Health, 33
Native American Church, 54
nightshade family, 55, 77. *See also*
    hallucinogens

opiates, 22, 85
  addiction to, 73–75
  mechanism of action, 72–73
  overdose, 72
  pain and, 72–74
  perceptual effects, 73–75
  physiological effects, 71–72
  psychological effects, 69–71, 74–75,
    86
optical illusions, 31. *See also*
    hallucinations
Osmond, Humphrey, 62

PCP (phencyclidine; Sernyl), 55
  deaths from, 78, 80
  history, 77–78
  medical uses, 77–78
  perceptual distortion from, 81–82
  physiologic effects, 80
  psychosis from, 78–79, 81–83

William A. Check is the author of *Drugs of the Future* in the ENCYCLOPEDIA OF PSYCHOACTIVE DRUGS SERIES 2 published by Chelsea House. He holds a Ph.D. in microbiology from Case Western Reserve University. He is the coauthor of *The Truth About AIDS* and a frequent contributor to medical reports for the National Institutes of Health and the Office of Technology Assessment.

Solomon H. Snyder, M.D., is Distinguished Service Professor of Neuroscience, Pharmacology and Psychiatry at The Johns Hopkins University School of Medicine. He has served as president of the Society for Neuroscience and in 1978 received the Albert Lasker Award in Medical Research. He has authored *Uses of Marijuana, Madness and the Brain, The Troubled Mind, Biological Aspects of Mental Disorder,* and edited *Perspective in Neuropharmacology: A Tribute to Julius Axelrod.* Professor Snyder was a research associate with Dr. Axelrod at the National Institutes of Health.

Barry L. Jacobs, Ph.D., is currently a professor in the program of neuroscience at Princeton University. Professor Jacobs is author of *Serotonin Neurotransmission and Behavior* and *Hallucinogens: Neurochemical, Behavioral and Clinical Perspectives.* He has written many journal articles in the field of neuroscience and contributed numerous chapters to books on behavior and brain science. He has been a member of several panels of the National Institute of Mental Health.

Joann Ellison Rodgers, M.S. (Columbia), became Deputy Director of Public Affairs and Director of Media Relations for the Johns Hopkins Medical Institutions in Baltimore, Maryland, in 1984 after 18 years as an award-winning science journalist and widely read columnist for the Hearst newspapers.